Path to Health

Path to Health

Where Science Meets Scripture

Susan Goe

XULON PRESS

Xulon Press
2301 Lucien Way #415
Maitland, FL 32751
407.339.4217
www.xulonpress.com

Printed in the United States of America.

Paperback ISBN-13: 978-1-6322-1632-8
Hardcover ISBN-13: 978-1-6322-1633-5
eBook ISBN-13: 978-1-6322-1634-2

Dedicated to my son
Christopher
October 21, 1970 – August 17, 1990

His ministry is his smile, his enthusiasm,
And his friendship.

Table of Contents

PREFACE

THIS WRITING PRESENTS SCIENTIFIC PROOF of the validity of biblical instruction for creating true health; the gold standard for living healthy and happy sitting right there on our coffee tables all along. The inability of so many Americans to mount an adequate immune response against the novel corona virus, during a recent pandemic, spotlights our already well documented poor state of health. The medical model is excellent for treating disease but, let us tell it like it is; this approach does little to improve our health. The time has come to address the crux of the problem; our ever-deteriorating pathologic lifestyles. It has been well known that "up to half of all premature deaths in the United States are due to behavioral and other preventable factors, including habits such as tobacco use, poor diet, and lack of exercise. Alcohol, opioids, and other drugs rank among the top offenders in impairing immunity and ruining the health of its victims. The psychological stress produced by guilt, resentment, social alienation, and reckless living drives upwards of eighty percent of physician visits." (National Research Council and Institute of Medicine report.)[1] Pouring more money on the current system has not worked.

Though the United States spends twice as much on health care per capita as other wealthy countries, our life expectancy is not only less but it is increasing at a slower rate.

I present you with fifty-two effective health promoting strategies, backed by medical and social sciences as well as by the Bible. We are blessed to be living in such a time as this when science is reconciling its findings and recommendations on best health practice with those described in the Bible for several thousand years. As a Disciple of Jesus, a seasoned health care provider, and a former health care administrator, I am well positioned to present these exciting findings to you. This book would be an excellent way for the more mature reader to evaluate and improve their current lifestyle practices but would also be a valuable gift to give to a truth seeking young person as a How to Live Healthy and Happy Manual.

I recommend that you initially scan through all fifty-two chapters. This will give you a flavor for the type and the scope of the proposed life changes and allow you to envision the genuine health you could expect should you decide to practice some or all of the strategies. You then might consider reading and incorporating several suggested practices into your own life at a rate of one chapter per week. The next year it would serve you well to then review, repeat or enhance each strategy. Some included strategies, such as diet, humor, and exercise will come as no surprise to you. Other, more esoteric strategies, such as purpose, identity, and trust, may surprise you by their inclusion but you will be pleasantly surprised by their impact on your health and happiness should you decide to embrace them. Each chapter includes both scientific and biblical perspectives as well as one of my no holes barred personal stories and a suggestion on how you might implement that particular strategy into your own life. My prayer is that your adoption of these strategies permeate your family and your community and result in health, happiness and peace for all.

DETOXIFY

What Science Says

HEADING TOWARDS THE DOWN SLOPE OF the first worldwide pandemic since 1918, the time is right to take a hard look at the effects of lifestyle on an individual's defense against opportunistic pathogens. COVID-19 has ravaged the world unabated and without regard for social status, ethnicity, religion, or political affiliation. It does, however, appear to raise more havoc in those with less robust immune systems, namely the elderly, and those with comorbidity. This variation in response is predictable, although it's presentation is inordinately more dramatic due to COVID-19's triple level of contagiousness and widely variable virulence. The vulnerability inherent in becoming elderly cannot be avoided but the burden of comorbidity can be greatly decreased. "It is known that "up to half of all premature deaths in the United States are due to behavioral and other preventable factors, including habits such as tobacco use, poor diet, and lack of exercise,"[1] according to studies reviewed in a National Research Council and Institute of Medicine report. "Alcohol, opioids, and other drugs rank among the top offenders in impairing immunity and ruining the health of its victims."[2] The psychological stress produced by guilt, resentment, social alienation, and reckless living drives upwards of eighty percent of physician visits. We could choose to perceive COVID-19 as a call to action, a time to ramp up our immunity and good health by changing the things we can change, namely our lifestyles. Like the first steps in remodeling a home involve the processes of planning followed by demolition and then rebuilding, so do the first steps in lifestyle change involve planning, detoxification and rebuilding. In both cases, removing the toxins precedes the rebuild. Just as the "big reveal" of a remodeled home elicits the admiration of a magnificent new structure, so does the detoxification and rebuild of an individual reveal a magnificent new life. The pandemic, horrific as it was, can be used as a bridge to a healthier, less toxic way of living. We are given an opportunity to change our diet and our exercise practice, and to eliminate drugs and excessive alcohol. We can use what we have gleaned from pandemic "stay at home" living to tamp down and modify our living choices. We could actually emerge from this scourge in history as a cleaner living, wiser, and more appreciative people; healthy and well positioned to face the next opportunistic viral or non viral threat that we will inevitably meet.

What God Says

God intended for us to treat our bodies with great care. "**Do you not know that you are God's temple**

and that God's Spirit dwells in you?" (Corinthians 3:16)[3] As with all direction from God, it bodes well for us to follow it, not so well if we choose not to. God knows that, having given us free will, we would need a way back from our inevitable poor choices. Once we have accepted God's offer of salvation and confessed and repented from our transgressions, His suffering for us on the cross, provides a way. "**If we confess our sins, He is faithful and just to forgive us our sins, and to cleanse us from all unrighteousness." (1 John 1:9)**[4] Confess and repent means that we see the error in our choices and and do an about face, desiring and determined to live life God's way. The more we do this, the closer we come to living healthy and strong; well positioned to face whatever threat the world throws our way. Whatever that threat might be, God promises us that he will **"work all things for good for those who love God and all called according to his purpose." (Romans 8:28)**[5]

One of My Stories

Once I felt secure that those I love were in a relatively safe position to ride out the COVID-19 pandemic, and was confident that the country's leadership was up to the challenge, I found myself profoundly interested in studying the ongoing response by the world to this sudden, unforeseen attack by an invisible, grievous enemy. Because I experienced the pandemic from a position of peace, my vantage point has been primarily one of ongoing fascination. I have been intrigued with studying the progression of the pandemic from the many perspectives; medical, societal, financial, political, and ethical. This comfortable stance would not have been possible twenty years ago. I would have felt defenseless and alone. Since accepting God's gift of salvation, I am privileged to depend on Him for wisdom and for strength. **"God is my refuge and strength, always ready to help in times of trouble."(Psalm 46:1)**[6] Over the years, I have applied that wisdom and strength to detoxify my lifestyle and to move towards a position of peace. God's Word has given me clear direction on diet, exercise, morality, simplicity, and peace of mind. It's been a revelation to me that the "gold standards" of health care that has developed and changed in the over fifty years that I have been in the medical field, has evolved to become the same as the Bible has been teaching for twenty three hundred years. My hope and my prayer is that you will use this lifestyle "pause" as an opportunity to detoxify and rebuild your life to one that is healthy, strong and able to weather the storms. For me, accepting God's invitation to join Him gives me a straight path to follow.

Write Your Story

Does the phrase "blessings in disguise" cause you to respond in fearful trepidation or optimistic anticipation? You do not have the option of choosing whether or not a COVID-19 pandemic, or any other major assault on your life, will occur, but what you can choose is how you will respond to it. Knowing the transformational effect that detoxification and rebuilding has had on my life and many others I know,

I am excited for you to have an opportunity for positive change. Going through a pandemic like experience can cause us to reevaluate priorities. If becoming physically and emotionally healthier rises to the top of your priority list, allow me to share what has worked for me. For starters, I get up and get moving. Walking or running has worked for me but whatever you enjoy doing is the right choice. Purge your cupboards of sugar, processed foods, cutting back on calories and alcohol and ramping up on fruits and vegetables. The next big step to work towards is living under your means. This could translate to a smaller house, an older car, less

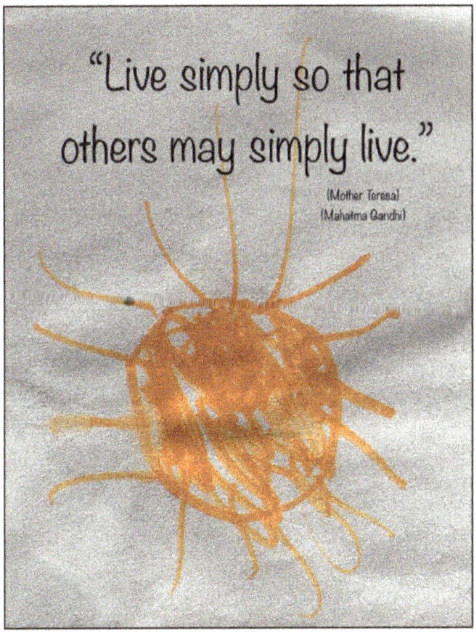

often going out, and more judicious spending . You might use a portion of the saved cash to set aside for the next "rainy day". Got any resentments, fears, or broken relationships? Address them. Solicit counseling when necessary. This is not easy but it is a must. What does your moral image look like, in terms of adhering to your standards? It is a great time to realign. If you need additional support in any of these areas, I am here to tell you that God is waiting with open arms. Now for the "big reveal". Picture this. If everyone decided, like you, to detoxify, simplify, and rebuild their lives, the total sum effect would be of global proportion. We would not only be happier, healthier individuals, we, as prudent stewards of earth, would "be living simply so that others could simply live."(Mother Teresa)(Mahatma Gandhi)[7]

Sunshine

What Science Says

Singer John Denver's hit song melodiously reminds us that "sunshine on our shoulders does make us happy." Here is how it works physiologically. Sunlight cues special areas in the retina, which triggers the release of serotonin, a feel good hormone. This, in turn, provides significant psychological benefits for the prevention and treatment of depression and anxiety related disorders. In addition, when our skin is exposed to sunlight, it makes vitamin D from cholesterol by providing the energy for vitamin D synthesis to occur. Vitamin D has proven effective in preventing multiple cancers, osteoporosis, cardiovascular diseases, and autoimmune disorders. A caveat to be considered, however, is that, in many urban areas, increased temperatures do translate to an increase in the amount of ozone produced, impacting negatively on people with lung disease such as asthma and COPD. Historically, sunshine has been effectively used as treatment for diseases such as tuberculosis, having a thirty percent improvement rate at sanatoriums. As with everything, sun exposure can be detrimental if done without discretion, the main risk being that of skin cancer. How much sun exposure, then, is needed for adequate vitamin D production without increasing the risk of skin cancer? Most conservative estimates are "about 15 minutes a day between 10 a.m. and 3 p.m., three times a week, depending on geographic latitude and personal skin color."[8] (Mayo Clinic). "As we head from north to south, latitudinally, we may find two or three extra deaths [per hundred thousand people] from skin cancer, while, at the same time, we will find thirty or forty fewer deaths for the other major cancers.[9] (Veith) As with most health recommendations, the answer lies in the correct balance. Consensus is to recommend getting outside to soak in some sunshine every day, while supplementing with the "sunshine vitamin," vitamin D, if sunshine is unavailable or inadequate. The positive sunshine effects may be compounded by adding play, socialization, and exercise, while avoiding over doing with sun burning and sporadic over and under exposure. Enjoyed with care, sunshine makes us happy and healthy.

What God Says

"Let there be light."[10] (Genesis 1:3) God created light on day one of creation, testimony in itself of it's importance to the world. In the Bible, light has always been a symbol of holiness, goodness, knowledge, wisdom, grace, hope, and God's revelation.

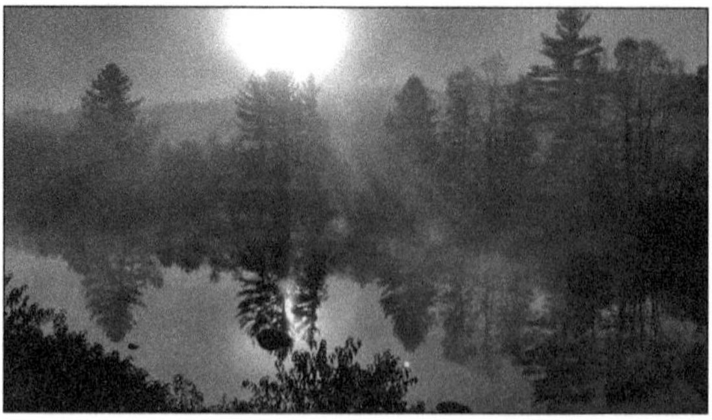

"I am the light of the world. The one who follows me will never walk in darkness, but will have the light of life."[11] (John 8:12) Metaphorically, when we "walk in the light," we live by the truth found in God's word. When we follow God's command to "love others" our hearts lead us to "shine our light" on those we love. **"No one lights a lamp and then covers it with a jar or puts it under a bed, but puts it on a lamp stand so that those who come in can see the light."**[12] **(Luke8:16-17)** The brilliant, life giving sun that gives life to the earth in the form of healthy warmth, light, and sustenance, can be a constant reminder of the "light giving" God who offers us His light, His truth and everlasting life.

One of My Stories

I, like most people I've known, have always been attracted to and affected by sunshine. With my contemporaries of the sixties, I baby oiled myself up and laid on the beach for hours to gain that movie star healthy look. Years later, as a healthcare provider, I rotely taught patients to stay out of the sun, use sun screen while in the sun, and take vitamin D supplements. Now, as a seasoned retrospective, I'm settled into spending as much time as possible having fun outdoors while avoiding burning or overdosing. Just thinking about going to visit my Tucson sibs, where it is sunny eighty five percent of the time, elevates my mood. Add sunshine to any activity, be it gardening, hiking, dining, or visiting and the enjoyment level is kicked up several notches. For me, since I have welcomed the Creator and His light into my heart, my life is spiritually illuminated. My prayer is that God uses me as a "lamp" through which His life light shines on others.

Write Your Story

Let the sun shine in; it is a gift, a gift that is most valuable when accepted with open arms and with gratitude. If you would like to use your radiant gift to improve your sleep, get up and go to bed as close to sunrise and sunset as possible. This causes your sun stimulated serotonin to convert to melatonin, allowing you to naturally and easily fall asleep. If a sunny outlook is what you're looking for, throw open the curtains and let the sun light permeate your space. If need be, use a light box during the short winter days. You can improve your health by going outside; walking, running, hiking, gardening, playing, or just standing there and soaking in the rays. Yes, do wear your sunscreen wisely and be careful not to overdo your exposure. As you quietly basque in the soothing warmth of the sun on your back, you may be inspired to contemplate it's Source.

Kindness

What Science Says

It's both contagious and addictive. It can be transmitted from person to person through intimate contact or simply by random observation. Just witnessing it causes the recipient to want to spread it to others. Fortunately, this communicable condition pervading certain niches in our country is kindness.

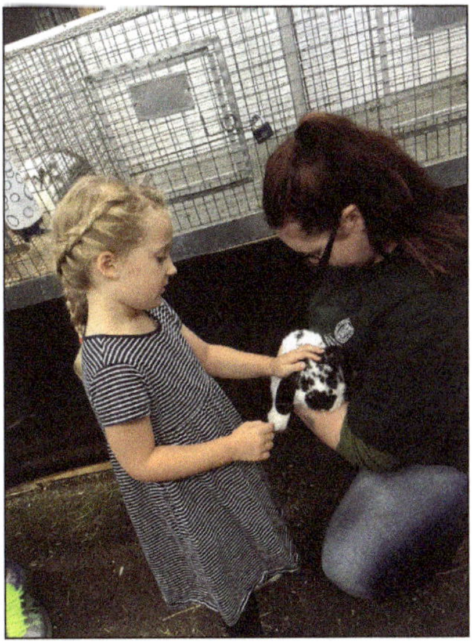

Seeing the symptoms and signs associated with kindness, schools and employers are creating environments and developing programs to encourage it's dissemination. Medical science has empirically demonstrated that kindness is good for one's health. Engaging in or even observing an act of kindness, such as inviting the new kid in school to join the group in the cafeteria, can cause the body of the doer, or even the observer, to produce the hormone, oxytocin. This hormone is effective in lowering blood pressure and increasing self-esteem. Inflammation is reduced with repetitive acts of kindness, thus reducing disease incidence.

What God Says

Kindness is mentioned and advocated for in the Bible hundreds of times. God prescribes the way to live a healthy life to his followers. **"Be kind to one another, tender-hearted, forgiving each other, just as God in Christ also has forgiven you."[13] (Ephesians 4:32.) Do not let kindness and truth leave you; Bind them around your neck, Write them on the tablet of your heart."[14] (Colossians 3:12)** Jesus, himself, in his time and culture, was perceived as a radical in his choice of people he demonstrated kindness to. He loved and provided healing to all, regardless of gender, social status or affiliations.

One of my Stories

I've recently been in a position to observe the effects of kindness in a virtual kindness oasis set amidst a less friendly world. My ninety two year old mom was placed in The Pines Nursing Facility for rehabilitation following surgical repair of a hip fracture. My sister and I were privileged to receive and to observe the positive effects of kindness on our mom's recovery. From receptionists to housekeepers, to caregivers, all treated us with engaged listening, warm smiles, and genuine compassion for the difficulty of the situation. We saw staff, at all levels, demonstrating the positive regard they had for each other and saw that positive energy filter down to the patients and the patients' families. It remains warmly fixed in my mind, an experience of observing a soft spoken lanky nursing assistant holding my mom's hand between his while accepting her gratitude for his care and adding that she was one of his faves. For myself, my sister, and for my mom, this greatly mediated the fears inherent in the situation.

Write Your Story

Each day offers new opportunity to improve one's physical, mental, and spiritual health through acts of kindness. Smile that smile, open that door for a stranger, give your focused time and attention to someone. Start with the lovable and work your way up to the more difficult to love. On day two, repeat day one. Then Wow! Bam! Notice the increase in your energy and your general happiness level. Watch out though. Kindness is highly contagious and will eventually infect those around you ultimately changing the world.

Diet

What Science Says

Our dietary choices are not only expanding our waistlines but they are responsible for most of our escalating national budget. 99% of the Medicare and 83% of the Medicaid budgets are the result of our poor dietary choices and the associated physical inactivity. It is predicted that one third of the children born after 2000 will develop diabetes in their lifetime. With autoimmune disorders and other chronic illnesses skyrocketing, medical science is scrutinizing the effects of diet on health. In our defense, we have been led astray by the seductive and highly addictive food choices presented to us. Even those of us who have looked to science for recommendations have been led astray. The Four Basic Food Group standard of the fifties was largely driven by the greed of the meat, dairy, and sugar industries. The Food Group Standard was subsequently improved and modified with the Food Pyramid. These were followed by MyPlate and currently the HealthyEatingPlate templates, but still finds us getting sicker. Disease reversing diets such as Paleo and Mediterranean diets are looking more and more like the diet originally created for man in the beginning and are demonstrating health improvement results.

What God Says

In the beginning, as God was preparing a paradise for His soon to be created man to enjoy and to flourish in, He spoke ideal foods into existence, **"And God said, Behold, I have given you every herb yielding seed, which is upon the face of all the earth, and every tree, in which is the fruit of a tree yielding seed; to you it shall be for food."[15] (Genesis 1:29)** These foods included fruits, vegetables and seeds. Much later, following sinful man's eviction from Paradise followed by the Flood wiping out most of the earth's inhabitants, God added certain meats as a dietary option. In the Biblical Book of Leviticus, one of God's many public health rules was to avoid disease causing animals such as camels and swine. He later cautions against overeating. ***"These are the regulations concerning animals, birds, every living thing that moves about in the water and every creature that moves along the ground. You must distinguish between the unclean and the clean, between living creatures that may be eaten and those that may not be eaten."[16] (Leviticus 11:46-47.) "Be not among drunkards or among gluttonous eaters of meat, for the drunkard and the glutton will come to poverty, and slumber will clothe them with rags."[17] (Proverbs 25:16)***

One of My Stories

Several years ago, after a beloved family member was diagnosed with Crohn's Disease, a chronic autoimmune disorder, in empathy with him, I made the decision to change to an inflammation reducing diet. I eliminated sugar, gluten, most dairy, processed foods and factory farm products while adding more fruits, vegetables and nuts. Within weeks, my eye and my skin rosacea symptoms were gone and I was able to stop the antibiotic I was on. Within six months my blood pressure lowered enough to stop a blood pressure medication. At seven months, I realized my irritable bowel symptoms had resolved. As a side benefit, I lost eight pounds, mostly belly fat. Sleep, energy, and cognition have improved. I was delighted in noticing that the foods I now eat mimic God's original diet.

Write Your Story

The good news is that every day you are offered a fresh start to improved health thru your dietary choices. I do realize that cheese fries and cinnabons are luring you in but trust that your desire for healthy foods will increase as you consistently and consciously choose them. This takes a few months but it will happen. Mark your calendar. It's all about perseverance. Consider purchasing a Mediterranean Diet, Paleo, Anti-inflammatory, or Autoimmune Cooking guide. Enjoy the food and enjoy your improved health. Please pass it on.

Purpose

What Science Says

WHAT THEY FOUND SHOCKED THEM, according to Celeste Leigh Pearce, one of the authors of the study published in JAMA Current Open. "People who didn't have a strong life purpose — which was defined as "a self-organizing life aim that stimulates goals — were more likely to die than those who did, and specifically more likely to die of cardiovascular diseases."[18] This association between a low level of purpose in life and death remained true despite how rich or poor participants were, and regardless of gender, race, or education level. The researchers also found the association to be so powerful that having a life purpose appeared to be more important for decreasing risk of death than drinking, smoking or exercising regularly. According to a 2017 Harvard Study, "positive health outcomes may be attributed to taking the focus off ourselves, which seems to be health-giving in more ways than one. Much of our mental anguish, stress and depression is linked to rumination and worry-based, self-referential thoughts. Transferring our focus from ourselves to another might work to quiet worry and distress about our own plight, much in the same way that meditation is known to quiet activity in the "me-centers" of the brain."[19]

What God Says

God, through His Word, directs us to lead our lives with purpose. **"God has given each of you some special abilities; be sure to use them to help each other, passing on to others God's many kinds of blessings."[20] (1Peter 4:10) "Live life with a due sense of responsibility, not as those who do not know the meaning of life but as those who do."[21] (Ephesians 5:15) "There are many plans in a person's mind, but it is the counsel of the Lord which will stand."[22] (Proverbs 19:21) "For we are his workmanship, having been created in Christ Jesus for good works that God prepared beforehand so we may do them."[23] (Ephesians 2:10)** Once again, science is concluding what God's Word has been telling us for thousands of years; living a life of purpose is the healthiest way to live. Pastor Rick Warren, in his best seller, "Purpose Driven Life," provides step by step instruction on how to lead a purposeful life. Three of the key principles are: 1. It's not about us, rather it's about service to others. 2. We are each suited for a special purpose based on our gifts, talents, and passions. 3. We are happier, healthier, and contribute more to the world if we align our lives with our gifts and passions.

One of my Stories

My Mom, Anna White, was purposed to serve through her gifts of nurturing, intelligence, and humor. As a young woman, she served her family of origin by earning income and caring for her younger siblings. She then chose to nurture her husband, her children, her grandchildren, and her great grandchildren by lovingly and exuberantly caring for their needs. In the midst of this, she also happily served customers, patients, and friends. As the years went by and family moved away, friends became ill or passed, and she was no longer employed, opportunity for nurturing became less and less. Then, about two years ago, while visiting my mom, mid work day, I casually mentioned to her that I was a little hungry. What was I thinking? I had just confessed to my Italian mother that I was hungry. Before I could take another a sip of coffee, the refrigerator door was flung open, mixing bowls were flying, the table was set, and the aroma of bacon frying and blueberry muffins baking filled the room. Not only did my mom again have a purpose, from that day forward, we got to share lunch, conversation, and a nap every work day. For the last few years, as her physical health was

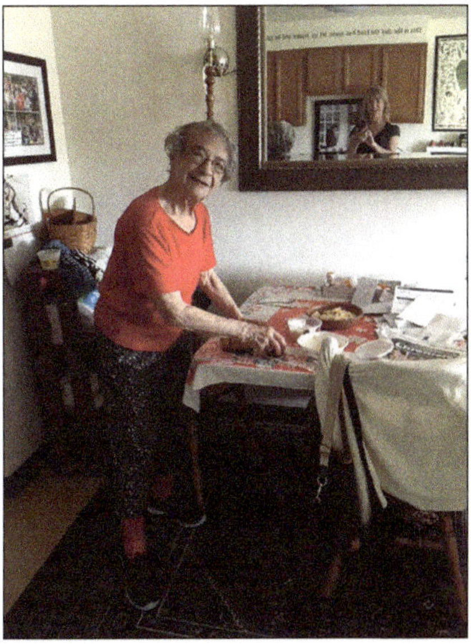

failing, she expressed frustration in not being able to do the kind of caring and nurturing acts she had always done but I witnessed her persevering in doing what she could do. She continued to contribute to family gatherings with her signature rice krispie cookies, and kept herself current with grandchildren activities by viewing my ipad photos and talking on the phone to family. We had opportunity to reminisce and pray in between. With extraordinary peace and in the knowledge that "she kept the faith and finished her course"(2Timothy 4:7), my mom, Anna G. White, passed September 25, 2019, from her temporary earthly residence to her eternal heavenly home. Surrounded by her family, her final words were, "I love you."

Write Your Story

You are not here by accident. You are perfectly and uniquely designed for a purpose and you will be healthier and more content if you figure out what that purpose is. As Pastor Rick Warren suggests, look at what things you're good at doing and what it is you could just love doing all day. You will probably need to talk with trusted friends or mentors for guidance and confirmation. If your aim is an over the top life adventure, throw a serving others goal into the equation. You could be looking at something vocational, voluntary, part time or even a variety of things. Test the waters. Talk, think, pray. No one else is qualified for your purpose.

What Science Says

Sit for a while in a room adorned with beautifully displayed Monet's or Renoir's and you will feel the healing effects of art. If you allow yourself to relax into the beauty, your blood pressure and pulse will decrease, and you will immerse in the moment with a few cleansing sighs. Art is defined as "the expression or application of human creative skill and imagination, typically in a visual form such as painting or sculpture, producing works to be appreciated primarily for

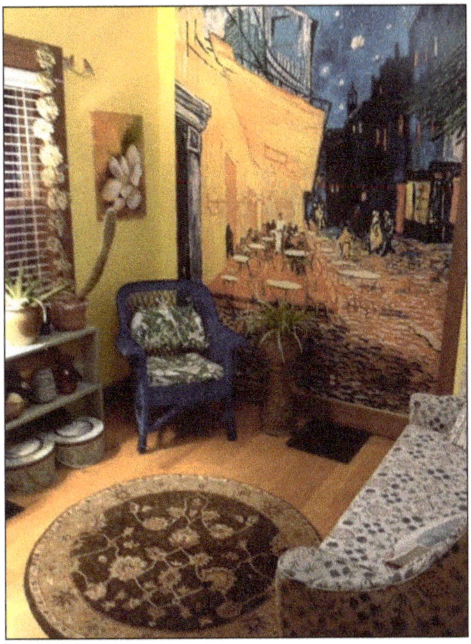

their beauty or emotional power." Research demonstrates that creative arts in healthcare can contribute to positive outcomes when services are integrated into medical treatment and community prevention and wellness programs. The research also demonstrates that art plays a role in improving socialization and maintaining an identity outside of the hospital. A study by Ercole Vellone and al. found that "among stroke survivors, those with interest in the arts enjoyed better general health, found it easier to walk, had more energy, and tended to be happier. They were also less likely to be depressed, or anxious. The results suggest that art may cause long term changes to the brain that help the person to recover when things go wrong."[24] The arts are also an aesthetically effective way to improve healthcare environments and benefit staff retention and professional development.

What God Says

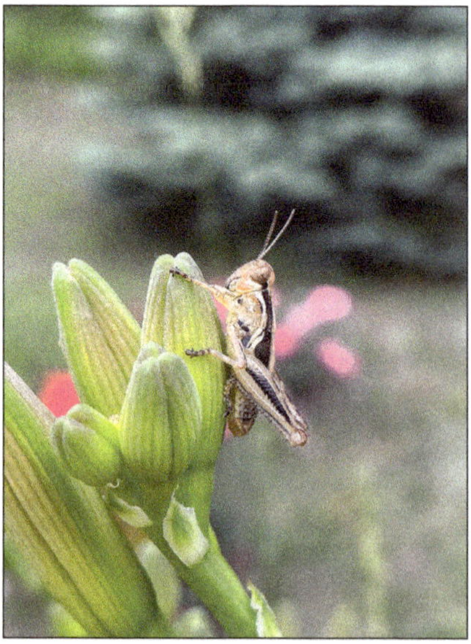

There is One who always was and always will be the primo artistic Creator of all, inspiring all other artists to capture even the slightest aspect of His divine design. Dante said it well, "Nature is the Art of God." Since God designed us "**in His image**," He incorporated a desire for Art in each of us. After each day of creation, God reflected on what He had made and evaluated it as good. At the end of the process, He declared it all to be very good. "**God saw all that he had made – and it was very good!"[25] (Genesis 1:31)**, the very first statement of art appreciation.

One of My Stories

I remain eternally grateful to God for the gift of having put in me a keen appreciation for art. I enjoy both God's created art through nature and man's art through various expressions of God's creation. From my point of view, the world is a perpetual art exhibit from the intricate structure and colors of a single flower to the breath taking panorama of the Adirondack Mountains. I find myself mesmerized by quietly laying face down on a dock starring at the bed of a lake or sitting on a rock examining a patch of the forest floor. It is sensory overload each time I visit my sister Tisha's dessert home where I am greeted by a whole new world of exotic art on display; cacti, red rock, and flat topped mesas. I am passionate about creating artful home respites to retreat to for myself or for any one else who invites me to. I am extraordinarily blessed to live in an area where I have opportunity to enjoy a four seasons portfolio of nature's art as well as artists' representation of the same.

Write Your Story

This is one of the few cases where instant gratification can be derived in a health promoting way. To begin, you might first try looking intentionally at a peaceful scene or at a painting you like. Contemplate the color, the lines, the textures and the shapes. Then, let your mood be changed by the over all message it conveys to you. Continue using this technique throughout your day to view faces, landscapes, buildings, and whatever else you encounter. "The world is your oyster." Use your increased sensitivity to broaden your enjoyment of your world through the lenses of an art connoisseur. You may just become a picture of health and happiness.

Giving

What Science Says

Be wary of a virulent contagion in our midst, predictably increasing it's effect every year around Christmas time. A study, published in the Proceedings of the National Academy of Science, shows that a highly contagious condition, "giving behaviors", can spread from one to dozens to hundreds of people, particularly during the Christmas season. To further compound it's effect, not only is "giving behaviors" contagious, it is also highly addictive. This condition, also referred to as "a helpers high," causes the addicted to want to give more and more. There is evidence that, "during giving behaviors, humans secrete "feel good" chemicals in their brains, such as serotonin, dopamine, and oxytocin (a compassion and bonding chemical)."[26] Many who succumb to this "giving" condition experience residual effects causing them to feel happier, have better social interactions, and have stronger immunity throughout the entire year. Stephen Post, a professor of preventative medicine at Stony Brook University, reports that "giving to others has been shown to increase health benefits in people with chronic illness, including HIV and multiple sclerosis."[27] It is well substantiated that, as this giving condition progresses, those affected become "carriers" potentially infecting many of their contacts, sometimes improving the health and happiness of entire communities. Givers, need to be informed and aware of the potential long term effects of their personal giving behaviors.

What God Says

There is no one in history who has come even close to out giving God. Since His goal for us while on this earth is to grow and flourish by becoming more like Him, He gives clear and repeated instruction about giving. "**It is more blessed to give than to receive.**"[28] **(Matthew 6:1-4)** Giving is not unlike any of the other biblical instructions to God's children, in that the giving benefits the giver as well as the receiver. **"A generous person will prosper; whoever refreshes others will be refreshed."[29] (Proverbs 11:25A).** The now popular "pay it forward" concept was first described in Matthew 18:21-35 in the story of a king's forgiveness of a slave's loan being carried forward to another slave. Benjamin Franklin, in a letter to Benjamin Webb dated April 25, 1784 again describes this same "paying it forward" concept as " a trick of mine for doing a great deal of good with a little money."[30] The Bible teaches us a method of receiving an even greater reward for our giving behavior; not letting anyone know what we did. **" But when you give to the needy, do not let your left hand know what your right hand is doing, so that your giving may be in secret. Then your Father, who sees what is done in secret, will reward you."[31] (Matthew 6:1-4)** By keeping our giving act a secret, not only do we then have a heavenly reward to look forward to, we get to hold the secret gift in our hearts, sometime making us feel like our hearts might burst.

One of My Stories

Tithing was my biggest leap of faith after which all subsequent leaps became easier. At a time in my life when my finances looked very bleak, I made the decision to have ten percent of my gross income automatically transferred from my checking account to my church's account. Contrary to what worldly advisers would have predicted, after two years, the color of my bottom line changed from red to black and there was an obvious upgrade in my own personal financial planning software. I have come to view money as a resource God has loaned me to use responsibly and generously. Because of it's limited supply, I see the resource of time as an even more valued treasure, reevaluating regularly how He would have me use it. I always keep in mind that **"For where my * treasure * is, there my heart will be also."[32] (Matthew 10:21)** Passing along what God has freely given me, and gift wrapping it in love, gives

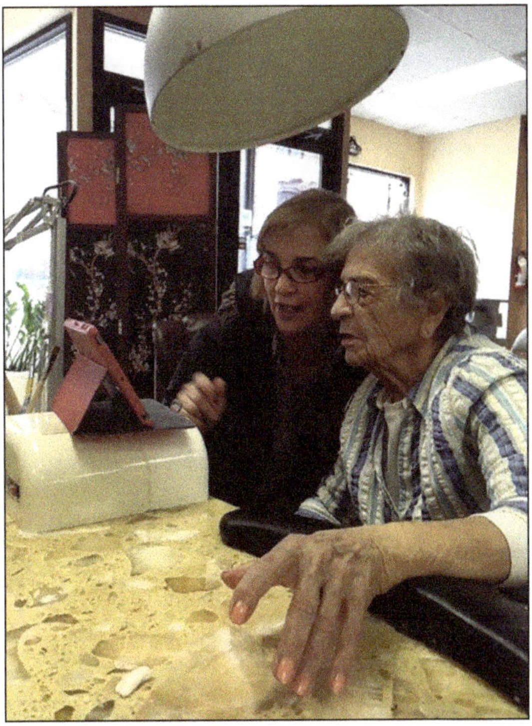

my life purpose, joy, and peace. One of the ways God directed me to spend extra time over the last several years was with my Mom. As her health started to fail, she and I would get together more often to shop, to have have manicures and to go to lunch. Although it was sometimes a challenge to find the time, the opportunities we did have to spend together and the memories of those experiences we shared will be forever sweet. I know that **"God loves a cheerful giver. And God is able to bless me abundantly, so that in all things at all times, having all that I need, I will abound in every good work."[33] (Psalm 112:5)**

Write Your Story

How to best spend your resource of money and your limited resource of time is a decision you make regularly and likely one of the more difficult. You either make your decisions decisively or you make them by default. If you want to look back, with minimal regret, on how you chose to use your resources, I gift you a plan that is working well for me. To begin, after much thought, meditation (I use prayer), and some consultation, record your four to five main life goals. Then develop your plan for achieving each of these goals, complete with time lines. Keep your plan accessible. Now you're ready for life to throw you choices. Say that, for example, that while walking in the mall, you notice a "buy one, get one half price" sale and that one of your goals is to be debt free in five years. Your closets are already bursting with clothes. You could quickly tell yourself, "Ou, ou, the more I buy, the more

I save," or you could consider your goals, go home, harvest your ripe closets and cheerfully give your surplus to a needy group; extra credit if you don't tell anyone what you did. How "in control" and "giving" would that make you feel? Anne Frank had it right, "No one has ever become poor by giving."[34] It does, in fact, lead to real wealth.

Exercise

What Science Says

Once upon a time, exercise was conveniently built into our daily routine. We walked to work and to school, tromped through the woods to hunt and fish for food, pounded our clothes and rugs and bread dough and more of us worked in occupations that were labor intensive. Children walked, ran, biked, climbed and rolled on a daily basis, both out of necessity and just for the fun of it. Though exercise is well proven to prevent disease, improve mood, enhance appearance, promote sleep, improve cognition and memory and even improve our sex lives, "only 22.9% of U.S. adults from ages 18 to 64 met 2008 guidelines for both aerobic and muscle-strengthening exercise between 2010 and 2015." (Centers for Disease Control and Prevention).[35] Currently, in order to build healthy exercise into our lives, we must be intentional. CDC recommends "at least 150 minutes a week of moderate aerobic activity, 75 minutes a week of vigorous aerobic activity, or a combination of moderate and vigorous activity."[36] The guidelines suggest that the exercise is spread throughout the week. Suggestions include running, walking or swimming. Even small amounts of physical activity are helpful, and accumulated activity throughout the day adds up to provide health benefits. Strength training exercises for all major muscle groups at least two times a week is additionally recommended. Examples include lifting free weights, using weight machines or doing body-weight training." It has been demonstrated that exercise becomes habit in about six weeks, during which time, Nike's "just do it" recommendation is efficacious.

What God Says

With exercise, as well as many other healthy practices, Jesus led by example. It is calculated that during his three year ministry Jesus and his apostles walked a total of 3,125 miles, averaging twenty miles per day. Also, thru his Word, God is consistent in his advocacy for our well being through his mention of exercise.

"A wise man is full of strength, and a man of knowledge enhances his might."[37] **(Proverbs 24:5)** Paul uses an athletic analogy again in **2 Timothy 4:7: "I have fought the good fight, I have finished the race, I have kept the faith."**[38] While the focus of these Scriptures is not on physical exercise, the fact that Paul uses athletic terminology to teach us spiritual truths indicates that Paul viewed physical exercise, and even competition, in a positive light. ***"So I do not run aimlessly; I do not box as one beating the air. But I discipline my body and keep it under control."***[39] **(1 Corinthians 9:26)**

One of my Stories

I have had the opportunity to observe the effects of exercise through several different lenses. As a "war crop" product, biking, running, and jumping was built into my childhood; no thought or planning required. I still can recall my exercise related pivotal day. Not long after giving birth to my third child, I was called to chase after one of them. I was surprised to find myself huffing and puffing, a heretofore foreign sensation. I stood at a crossroads; continue my life of relative inertia and huff and puff with exertion or intentionally start exercising. I exercised in the house and in the wood, and in the gym whenever I could. I ran alone. I ran for fun. I danced and hiked with everyone. As both a family member and a health care provider, I've been privileged to witness the health of those I care about and care for improve, even soar, partly as a result of my sharing my knowledge, experience and zest for exercise. Currently I'm settled into a regime of walkin 'n talkin in the morning with strengthening with weights to the rhythm of my husband's drumming later in the day. Hiking, skiing, kayaking and landscaping are among my fun substitutions.

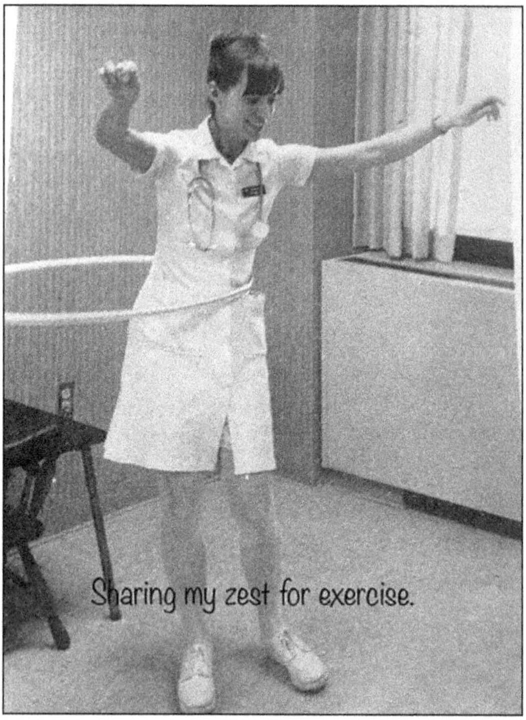

Sharing my zest for exercise.

Write Your Story

Few would argue that exercise is health enhancing. Happily, any amount or type of exercise is beneficial, done consecutively or done incrementally. It can be high impact or it can be low, done with a friend or done on the go. The best choice is exercise that you will do. Give some serious thought about what you might enjoy or learn to enjoy doing. The options are limitless from playing tag in the pool with your kids to training for a marathon. Walking up flights of stairs at work when added to briskly walking the dog and stacking the wood can be as effective as a work out at the gym using a treadmill and free weights. It's all about persistence and creativity with a touch of whimsy added for fun. You've got what it takes. So it's one, two, three, four, put on your sneaks and walk out the door.

COMPETENCE

What Science Says

"COMPETENCE IS THE REQUIRED SKILL, knowledge, qualification, or capacity for our specified work or situation."[40] (Kathy Koch PhD) "We are born with an inherent tendency to want to develop ourselves. This means that we actively strive to become effective, to master our environments, and to hone our capacities in order to reach our innate potential."[41] (Deci and Ryan 2002; Harter 1983) Competence is not only crucial for building self-esteem, it is also integral in acquiring health promoting activities such as bike riding or playing tennis. Acquiring competence in any endeavor requires that infamous, often fear provoking, first step; the first stride of a run, the first pedal to the metal of a bike ride or the first step-tap-step of a ballroom dance. As we become more skilled at a task, our confidence grows but herein lies the rub; how to possess sufficient confidence to take that first step. The same techniques that parents and teachers employ to spiral competence, and the resultant confidence in children, can be successfully used in any mentoring situation, including self-mentoring. "Competence, not perfection, is the goal. Instead of pointing out mistakes as problems, we should encourage those we mentor to make mistakes in order to get better. We should point out how we have learned from our own mistakes. We can discourage negative self-talk by modeling positive self-talk about ourselves and about others. The more positive messages are heard about oneself and about others, the more a person will internalize positive self-talk in his own mind."[42] (Holistic Child Psychologist, Dr. Nicole Beurkens) "Perceptions of competence are said to be just as important for success as actual competence. Observers evaluated those who made optimistic predictions as much more competent than their modest contemporaries, no matter how accurate those predictions were and how well they actually performed. This seems to suggest that if someone asks us how we expect to perform, we should give a positive, confident response. As we become more skilled at one task, our fears shrink and our confidence grows. As our confidence grows, we become more competent."[43] (Psychologists Barry Schlenker and Mark Leary) Competencies are like building blocks. Once we gain competencies in a couple areas, despite the initial fear and inevitable mistakes, we are more prepared to embrace subsequent challenges.

What God Says

Followers of Christ have God's Word that he will provide unlimited strength and support in securing the competencies required to fulfill their life's purpose. God promises His children that, **"I can do all things**

through Christ who strengthens me."[44] (Philippians 4:13) When going through a difficult time, children of God can be secure in tapping into God's supreme power, **"I am strong in the Lord and in the power of His might."(Ephesians 6:19)** By accepting God's invitation to be a member of His family, Christians have direct access to a divine loving Father and can know that **"I can approach God with freedom and confidence."[45] (Ephesians 3:12)** With the loving backing of God the Father, competencies may be achieved with divine confidence.

One of My Stories

Preparing to address a large group of strong spirited nurses for whom I was the newly hired director, I replaced the "run" tape in the forefront of my mind with a past tape of me enthusiastically leading a large aerobics class. In the tape, the music was rhythmic, and my voice strong and confident, the result of having led many classes. I had subconsciously developed this habit of giving myself a therapeutic injection of confidence related to past competencies whenever I faced that first step in learning a new competency. I believe I owe this habit, at least in part, to the wise practice of the Girl Scouts of America in rewarding with colorful badges for each competency achieved, whether it be sewing, selling cookies, or marching in form in a parade. The ceremonial receiving of the badge and the displaying of it on my Girl Scout sash served to remind me and others that, yes, I was capable of being competent. Each subsequent step out, despite the ever present fear factor, fell into an increasingly more comfortable pattern; desire to become competent at something and recollection of past successes. This was followed by trials and errors and ultimately successes, considering that a decisive change in course also qualifies as a success. I would be remiss in not mentioning that, since I have accepted God's invitation to be part of his family, I can call on Him for whatever I might be lacking, remembering that **"I can do all things through Christ who strengthens me."[46] (Philippians 4:13)**

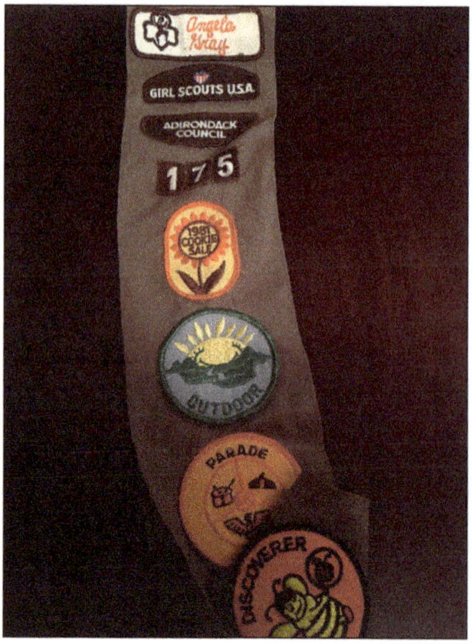

Write Your Story

The desire to do well, to become competent, is in you. Developing competencies is unquestionably good for your spiritual, your emotional and your physical health. Everything you need to develop competencies, you already possess or it is available to you. Say you have always had a burning desire to bake a consistently delicious and attractive apple pie. Notice I did not say "perfect." Start with positive self-talk and recollection of a past competency. The past competency may be related or unrelated to the situation at hand. Remember, for example, how your Aunt Julia raved about the strawberry shortcake you made for last year's family reunion. Now step out and do the work part with all the confidence you have gleaned from your past. This step might involve, recipe research, conversations with good bakers you know, and even a few trial and error learning experiences. Ultimately, voila, la piece de resistance. Bring on the pie. Shore up your confidence bank with this new competency and exuberantly bring on the the next opportunity to grow. Be like Thomas, "I have not failed. I've just found 10,000 ways that won't work."[47] (Thomas Edison)

Nature

What Science Says

Go take a hike! Medical science is accruing more and more evidence to support this aphorism as an effective medical prescription. A group of Outward Bound participants, for example, scored an astounding 50 percent higher on creative problem-solving tasks after three days of wilderness backpacking. Another health enhancing option is forest bathing or Shinrin-yoku; simply soaking up the sights, smells, and sounds of nature. This increasingly popular revived Japanese practice has been proven to reduce blood pressure, lower blood sugars, and improve energy. Other recent studies have found that spending time in, or living close to natural green spaces is associated with reducing the risk of type II diabetes, cardiovascular disease, premature death, and preterm birth, while increasing sleep duration and decreasing levels of salivary cortisol, a physiologic marker of stress.

What God Says

In the beginning, God the Father chose to place his newly created man and woman in a garden, a beautiful place he had previously created, perfectly designed for their health and happiness. **"The Lord God made all kinds of trees grow out of the ground—trees that were pleasing to the eye and good for food. The Lord God took the man and put him in the garden**

of Eden to work it and keep it."[48] (Genesis 2:15) Later God comforts us with the imagery of the 23rd psalm, **"He makes me lie down in green pastures. He leads me beside still waters.[49] (Psalm 23:2)** Forest bathing and nature therapies were introduced.

One of My Stories

Mud Creek exploring, picking wild berries in the fields, designing leaf houses, and climbing into tree forts are among my fondest childhood memories. Every waking minute I could, I was drawn to the rich fragrances of fresh grasses, wild strawberries, and various woods. I still recall the feel of mud beneath my sneakers and the creek water seeping in when I needed to get closer for a better look. The bright oranges and yellows of wild flowers against the various greens and browns of the fields and trees were so easy on my eyes. The sun on my face while laying in the tall grass and hearing the birds and peepers singing is a sensation I still attempt to replicate. At the time, I did not realize that nature was supplying every one of my senses with a lovely array of gifts,

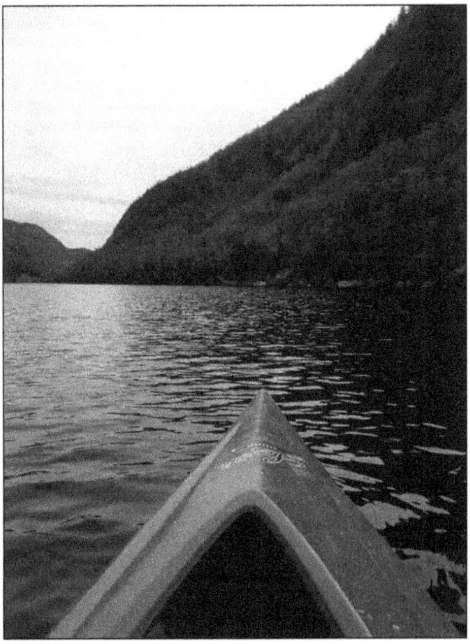

causing me to feel both happy and peaceful. Attempting to recreate this feeling, I still lay on my back in a field with sun on my face whenever possible. I have also learned to achieve that peaceful easy feeling in many other ways. Taking a hike or a ski through the Adirondack woods or trekking up a mountain leaves me feeling refreshed and restored with an enlightened perspective on life. If you see me out there, I'll be the one saying, "thank you God for your spectacular creation and for giving me the ability to be out here." Just thanking Him kicks the already great feeling up a few more notches.

Write Your Story

At last, a prescription that is good for your health and fun too. There are so many wonderful options for improving your health through communing with nature; a hike in the woods, eating lunch in the park, planting trees and plants around your house or walking in your neighborhood are just a few ideas. If you are in a city, taking walks in the park and displaying lots of green plants in your apartment also works. Your senses deserve a treat today. Soak in the sights, and the sounds. Take deep breaths. Enjoy with a friend or go solo. I will see you out there.

Service

What Science Says

The greatest leaders and humanitarians, throughout the ages, have advocated that we serve others. To serve is for the good of the world, for the good of the country, for the good of the community and for the good of the server. The Greek philosopher, Aristotle, once surmised that the essence of life is "To serve others and do good."[50] Benjamin Franklin's philosophy was "one served not to save their soul, but to build a strong society."[51] Martin Luther King Jr said in 1957, "Life's most persistent and urgent question is, 'What are you doing for others?"[52] Most recently, John F. Kennedy rocked the country with this section of his Inaugural Address, "And so, my fellow Americans: ask not what your country can do for you — ask what you can do for your country. My fellow citizens of the world: ask not what America will do for you, but what together we can do for the freedom of man."[53] Evidence of volunteerism's physical effects on the volunteer can be found in a study from Carnegie Mellon University, published in Psychology and Aging. "Adults over age 50 who volunteered on a regular basis were less likely to develop high blood pressure than non-volunteers."[54] This is significant because high blood pressure is an important indicator of health. It contributes to heart disease, stroke, and premature death. Volunteering is also excellent for the psychological health of our young people. Experience has shown that "teens who volunteer are 50% less likely to participate in risky behaviors, are less likely to become pregnant and use drugs, and are more likely to experience psychological well-being. It is also found that teens are very good at serving." According to research, "young people are well-suited to solve complicated social problems. Between the ages of 12 and 25, when their brains are fast and sophisticated, teenagers and young adults are especially wired to seek new experiences and take risks. It is important to note that, at all levels of maturity, one key for deriving health benefits from volunteering is to do it for the right reasons." A 2012 study in the Journal of Health Psychology found that "participants who volunteered with some regularity lived longer, but only if their intentions were truly altruistic. In other words, they had to be volunteering to help others—not to make themselves feel better."[55] In addition to improvement in health, the benefits of volunteering our service are many; increasing social opportunity, making job connections, skill development, resume building, and providing for very real needs, just to name a few. I would suspect that, even if our motives for volunteering may be partially self serving initially, once we experience the positive effects it has on others, our compassion and altruism will grow.

What God Says

When it comes to serving, Jesus was consistent and concise. **"It is more blessed to give than to receive."[56] (Acts 20:35)** When answering the question as to how to be the greatest, Jesus amazed his listeners with, "**Whoever wants to become great among you must be your servant, and whoever wants to be first must be your slave.**"[57] **(Matthew 20:26-28)** "**Do nothing out of selfish ambition or vain conceit. Rather, in humility, value others above yourselves, not looking to your own interests but each of you to the interests of the others.**"[58] **(Philippians 2:3-4)** When asked about who we should serve, Jesus responded with the often cited parable of the Good Samaritan, telling us that we are to serve even our enemies. God's commands, though often a paradox by world standards, are always met for our personal good and the good of mankind. Our loving Father also addresses any skepticism we might have about about our abilities to provide the service he has led us to. The Bible assures us, **"For we are God's masterpiece. He has created us anew in Christ Jesus, so we can do the good things he planned for us long ago"**[59] **(Ephesians 2:19)** Jesus, to the consternation of his disciples, defied the cultural tradition of his day, by washing the feet of his disciples, and healing lepers, tax collectors and other untouchables. Those of us who embrace God's inverted worldly paradigm, are privileged to reap the rewards of living as servants, even in this world, knowing from scripture and also in our hearts that we should not look to our own interests but to the interest of others.

One of my Stories

I was not surprised to learn that the greatest number of the thirty percent of Americans who volunteer are the people with the least amount of discretionary time; working moms. A stellar example of this is my beautiful Aunt Rose. She was able to orchestrate running a household, raising four children, caring for parents, and working a job while volunteering to serve others. She was the first to volunteer in preparing exquisite Italian dishes for her church, the rescue squad or any group that asked her. She also said yes to teaching catechism class to rambunctious after schoolers and serving the community through her church's Ladies of Mt. Carmel. Most memorable about my Aunt Rose was that, whoever she served, myself included, received a generous portion of her love and caring. On the other side of the generation line is my daughter Angela; different time, similar scenario, just replace the cooking with scholastics and athletics. The future looks bright with volunteering already being practiced by her children.

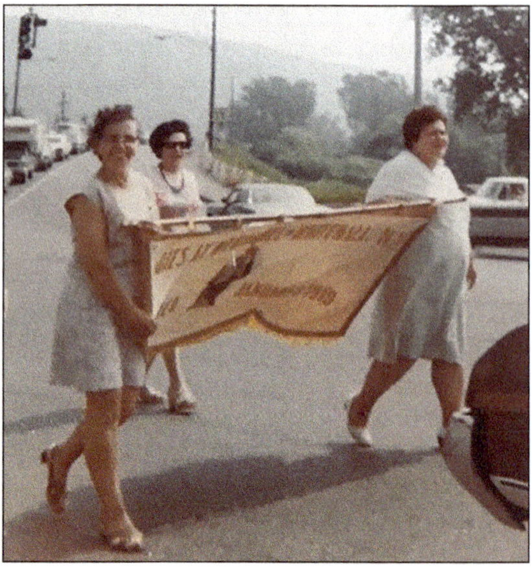

Write Your Story

Jump on a bandwagon. You will love the ride. You can ride nationally, locally, with a small group or on a one on one basis. On the national front, you could join or donate to Samaritan's Purse, a charitable christian team who mobilize with staff, equipment and thousands of volunteers to provide emergency aid to victims of tornadoes, hurricanes, wildfires, floods, and other natural disasters in the United States, currently responding to a crisis in Tennessee. On the local front, you could have joined over eight hundred middle and high school students from South Glens Falls, a local school, who, with strong community support, danced their hearts out for the forty third year to raise money to help individuals in need. Small group options include helping to lead youth groups at your church or school or, on a smaller scale, you could volunteer your time to read to preschool children or nursing home residents. Find the service that suits you and jump on the band wagon. You may just find that, "The best way to find yourself is to lose yourself in the service of others."[60] (Mahatma Gandhi)

Breathe

What Science Says

Inhale the good air in. Exhale the bad air out. Sounds quite simple but even this basic life process has options. Diaphragmatic breathing, for instance, comes from the body's dominant breathing muscle, the diaphragm. This type of breathing is the most effective and efficient. It can lead to feelings of relaxation instead of tightness. Chest breathing, on the other hand, which uses secondary muscles in the upper chest, is physiologically designed to be used in situations of great exertion, such as a sprinting in a race or in times of real or perceived danger. Unintentionally holding your breath during a stressful moment, even for as small a provocation as reading an upsetting email, can likewise distress your body. According to Belisa Vranich Ph.D.,author of "Breathing Technique," "three out of ten people have unintentional breath holding episodes daily."[61] Chest Breathing can lead to tight shoulder and neck muscles and sometimes even headaches. If one is chronically stressed, these symptoms will be magnified. "During stressful moments, consciously breathing diaphragmatically can allow you to shift and release negative energy instead of storing it in your body. Breathing diaphragmatically is especially significant with chronic breathing conditions such as asthma and COPD, where, over time, chest breathing leads to air being trapped in the lungs, causing them to lose their effectiveness."[62] (American

Lung Association) There is solution. It is free and it comes standard with your body, no extra equipment required. Diaphragmatic breathing can be used preventively, or therapeutically. "It is one of the best ways to lower stress because when you breathe deeply, it sends a message to your brain to calm down and relax. The brain then sends this message to your body. Those things that happen when you are stressed, such as increased heart rate, fast breathing, and high blood pressure, all decrease as you breathe diaphragmatically. There are a wide variety of breathing methods described. Diaphragmatic breathing is basic and highly effective.

What God Says

In the Bible's creation story, "Breath" is equated to "life". **"Then the LORD God formed a man from the dust of the ground and breathed into his nostrils the breath of life, and the man became a living being."[63] (Genesis 2:7)** Breath is used metaphorically to compare the imperative of breathing for man's physical life, to the need for scripture for mankind's spiritual, emotional, and physical life. "**Scripture is breathed out by God and profitable for teaching, for reproof, for correction, and for training in righteousness, that the man of God may be competent, equipped for every good work."[64] (2Timothy 3:16-17)** Like intentional deep breathing, "spiritual breathing is an exercise in faith that enables us to experience God's love and forgiveness and walk in the Spirit."[65] (Bill Bright, founder of Campus Crusade for

Christ) Spiritual breathing is something that requires conscious action; an exhale of our sins and an inhale of The Holy Spirit, another "out with the bad and in with the good," healing not only our physical self but, more importantly, our spiritual self as well. Jesus modeled the ultimate cleansing breath for us in dying for forgiveness of our sins. **"Father, into your hands I commit my spirit! " And after he said this he breathed his last.[66] (Luke 23:46)**

One of My Stories

The patient presents with a history of squeezing chest pain with shortness of breath, increasing in frequency, intensity and duration. Call the rescue squad. No, wait. It's me, me who feels way better running on the bike trail than sitting on the couch. Over the course of six months, as life stressors waxed and waned, my chest pain and other related symptoms were evaluated with lab tests, physical exams, allergy testing and heart and lung work ups. I was treated with pills, immunotherapy, inhalers, and eye drops, while continuing to exercise, eat healthy and avoid known toxins. Tests were all normal. Interventions were ineffective. I prayed about it, handed it over to God and thanked Him in advance for good health. A few days later, over a cup of ginger/turmeric tea, I asked my daughter, Angela, "What do you think would be a good topic for my next health blog?" "Breathing," she quickly came back with. "Super idea," I said. I did my research on breathing, while continuing my research on chest pain causes. Then, Eureka. The two research paths crossed. I diagnosed myself with anxiety attacks and started diaphragmatic breathing at a rate of several sets of ten repetition per day, adding an additional few breaths whenever stress was high. Within one week, the chest pain was gone. I do disclose that my practice of diaphragmatic breathing incorporated exhaling my worries to God's control and inhaling the Holy Spirit to guide me. I believe this complement likely positively skewed the results in my favor.

Write Your Story

What if you were told that there is something that is simple to learn, helps you sleep, makes you feel relaxed, and makes you healthier. Oh, and it's free and can be done anywhere, any time? This is a gift that, once you master it, you can practice daily to maintain your peace or as needed when you meet one of those bumps in your day. There is also the option of combining it with Yoga and Meditation or Music. Ready? Here it is. Breathe in. Breathe out. Repeat. (See illustration) Until you try it consistently, you will be not believe the very positive effects of deep diaphragmatic breathing on your health and well being. "When you own your breath, no one can steal your peace."[67] (Unknown author)

Diaphragmatic Breathing Technique

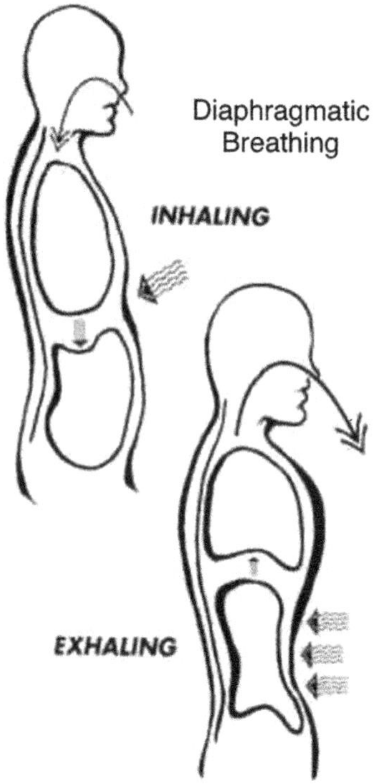

Diaphragmatic Breathing Technique

Place one hand on your upper chest and the other Just below your rib cage.
This will allow you to feel your diaphragm move as you breathe.
Breathe in slowly through your nose so that your stomach moves out against your hand.
The hand on your chest should remain as still as possible.
Then breathe out, fully emptying your lungs, while causing your stomach to pull in. (Cleveland Clinic)

FAMILY

What Science Says

"THE FAMILY IS THE BUILDING BLOCK OF society. It is a nursery, a school, a hospital, a leisure center, a place of refuge, and a place of rest."[68] (Margaret Thatcher, former Prime Minister U.K.) This assertion is supported by study after study indicating that strong families with a married biological mother and father are the best environment for rearing children. Theodore Roosevelt broadened these findings in declaring that, "Strong nations are built out of strong families, not the other way around."[69] Although, in surveys, Americans today describe family relations as the most meaningful part of their lives, far surpassing work and friends, in the past fifty years, the number and the cohesiveness of American families has taken a drastic plunge to the extreme detriment of the country. In 1970, eighty four percent of U.S. children spent their entire childhoods living with both bio-parents. Today, only half can expect to do the same. These downward trends in family structure is attributed to multiple societal changes, the launching of the sexual revolution through the advent of "the pill" being most significant. The pervasive choice to cohabitate prior to, or instead of, marriage, has resulted in four times the family dissolution rate."[70] (Osborne, Manning, and Stock 2007).

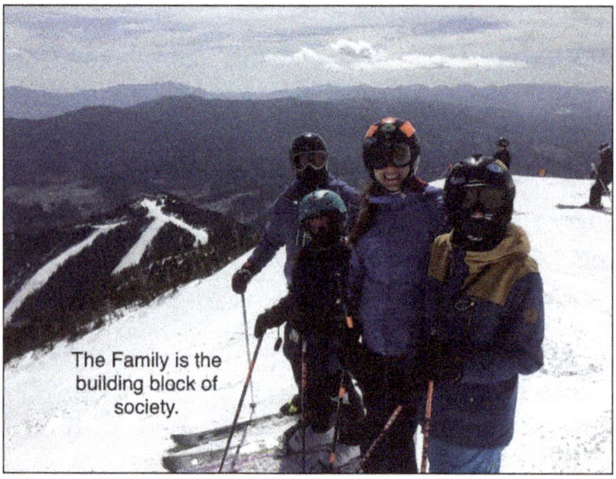

Adults and children in single-parent households are at risk for adverse health outcomes, including mental illness (e.g. substance abuse, depression, suicide) and unhealthy behaviors (e.g. smoking, excessive alcohol use, food insecurity). The nuclear family, "the building block of society," continues to be crushed from multiple fronts. The media, for instance, has gone from "Father Knows Best's" depiction of a caring strong father of the fifties to the current portrayal of a bumbling doofus dad in shows such as TV's Homer Simpson. "Legislation of 1986, as part of the War on Drug effort, though well intended, led to mass incarceration and the collapse of lower socioeconomic nuclear families, disproportionally effecting blacks."[71] (Patrick Moynihan Report) What can we do to turn around this demise of family? There are actions we as individuals and as a society can take. In terms of legislation, on December 21, 2018, the president signed into law the First Step Act. This legislation reformed sentencing laws that had "wrongly and disproportionately harmed the African-American community." This new law gives nonviolent criminals, including many dads, the chance to reenter the workforce and join their nuclear family. Additionally, laws, giving leave time to new parents and the FMLA (Family Medical Leave Act) have been enacted to assist in family survival. Employers, recognizing the value of intact and happy families to their bottom line, support families through onsite day care, flexible scheduling, and work at home options. The education system could support families more by increasing curricula on the value and dynamics of family and by teaching basic relationship and home management skills. As individuals, we can show respect for the family by avoiding media and advertised products that deride and mock family members. We can also demonstrate support for our own and other families through honoring fidelity. The church offers biblical support, child education, and community and marital education in recognition of the value of the family. Quoting the pastor and renown author Max Lucado, "They call them Mom. They call them Dad. And these moms and dads, more valuable than all the executives and lawmakers west of the Mississippi, quietly hold the world together."[72]

What God Says

God's commands are always intended for our good and His direction regarding family is no exception. Not long after creating Adam, God created Eve so that Adam would not be alone, uniting them "**in one flesh**" and extorting them ""**be fruitful and multiply"**[73] **(Genesis 1:22)**, thus the formation of the original "first family." The family is so important to God that He gives every member clear instruction. **"Husbands, love your wives, just as Christ loved the church and gave himself up for her."**[74] **(Ephesians 5:25) "Likewise, wives, be subject to your own husbands, so that even if some do not obey the word, they may be won without a word by the conduct of their wives."**[75] **(1Peter 3:1)** To dads, **"Fathers, do not provoke your children to anger by the way you treat them. Rather, bring them up with the discipline and instruction that comes from the Lord."**[76] **(Ephesians 6:4)** To both parents, "**Train a child in the way that he should go, and when he is old he will not turn from it."**[77] **(Proverbs 22:6)** Children are instructed, **"Honor your father and mother, and love your neighbor as yourself."**[78] **(Matthew 19:19)** God recognizes the sanctity of the marriage in consistently denouncing adultery. **"Thou shall not commit adultery."**[79] **(Exodus 20:14).** God entrusts care to the family, including the extended family, **"But if anyone does not provide for his relatives, and especially for members of his household, he has denied the faith and is worse than an unbeliever.**[80] **(1 Timothy 5:8).** Society at large is mandated to support family, **"Therefore what God has joined together, let no one separate."**[81] **(Mark 10:9)**

One of My Stories

As a member of the fraternal order of dysfunctional American families, I am in good company with membership comprising seventy to eighty percent of the American population. I will, however, be eternally grateful for my kinship status, qualifying me for life long access to unconditional love and acceptance, community support, and companionship. With a background of family of origin dysfunction due to alcohol, and while, at the same time, living within a society whose values had shifted from family to individual fulfillment, I unwittingly allowed myself to be ruled by feelings, and made decisions that led to the dissolution of my nuclear family. In retrospect, these were the most tragic decisions of my life. From the, now, vantage point of having been formally educated, and having had the benefits of observation and experience, I perceive the nuclear and the extended family as, not only valuable, but essential. I am grateful and hopeful whenever I see societal, governmental, ecclesiastical, or individual support of the family. The sediment that "your

fam is your jam," expressed and practiced by some of the current generation brightens my view of the future. Everyone has within them the desire to belong and family membership is the natural and healthy way to fulfill this need. Want world peace, look to family; created by God and promoted by healthy societies. Mother Theresa wisely summed it up, "What can you do to promote world peace? Go home and love your family."[82]

Write Your Story

If you are a young person thinking about your options for a permanent living arrangement, strongly consider the nuclear family; father, mother, and children. It is a time tested model proven proficient in providing the human need for belonging while creating the research backed environment for your optimal health. Additionally, family provides for financial stability, sexual fulfillment, and, not to forget to mention, it propagates the species. If you are lacking in positive family experience, successful family life is still feasible but will, like anything else you lack expertise in, require education and wise counsel. I suggest you reject provocative worldly advise to just cohabitate to test it out, or to pursue free love (lust) rather than to limit yourself to one sexual partner. Both science and scripture support the folly in these options. If you are already a member of a family and are running into difficulties, for the sake of the happiness of every family member, go to any length to reach resolution. Extended family members; support your young, very busy nuclear families. Young families; engage and involve extended family, maintaining a high threshold for being offended and mending relationships as they occur. Everyone wins. If nuclear family life is not for you, look for opportunity to be more involved with your extended family, or a church family. If you have been blessed with a harmonious family life, why not enhance it by reaching out individually, or through an organization, to help the disenfranchised? Keep in mind that someday you may enjoy a divine membership in the family of God the Father. Would it not be desirable to be already known by a variety of your new siblings?

Humor

What Science Says

Rx: One good belly laugh every two hours. Norman Cousins is renowned for having brought attention to the effects of laughter on healing and pain relief. By watching the comedian Groucho Mark's movies, Cousins healed himself from a painful, dismally prognosed illness after conventional medicine had failed. Science has proven the effects of laughter and humor on the body through the measurement of healing and pain relieving chemicals such as endorphins, and dopamine. Multiple subsequent studies support these findings.

What God Says

The importance of humor to a healthy life is repeated throughout the Bible.

"A cheerful heart is good medicine, but a crushed spirit dries up the bones."[83] (Proverbs 17:22) "He that is of a merry heart has a continual feast."[84] (Proverbs 15:15) Jesus often used humor in his teachings. **"Better to live on a corner of the roof than share a house with a quarrelsome wife."[85] (Proverbs 25:2)** It's difficult to forget His message about marriage with this vision in mind, He also used an effective visual analogy to point out the hypocrisy in judging others. **"Why do you look at a splinter**

from from your eye while you have a log in your own."[86] (Matthew 7:5)

One of My Stories

I walked into the hospital cafeteria having recently broken up with my long term boyfriend and there he was, for all to see, sitting cozily with his new squeeze. I was faced with the decision of where to put down my tray of iceberg lettuce and pseudo ice cream. To the left was the Debbie Downer table, more than ready to support me in justifying my feelings of rejection and pain. Quickly searching for an alternative, my eyes were drawn to the table to right. There was animation and laughter. I had never sat with this group but felt a desperate need for a dose of what they had. They welcomed me in and before lunch was over, I was laughing, the heaviness in my body and in my heart had lightened and my perspective had broadened. Though thirty years ago, the effects of my table choice was so profound that it remains at the forefront of my memory.

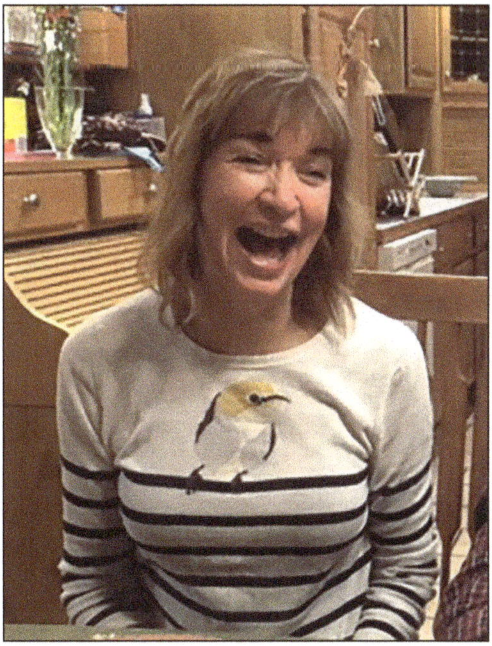

Write Your Story

Knowing that incorporating humor into your life is both preventative and restorative, how might you improve on your current sense of humor and use it to approach your next life challenge? You might have fun by arming yourself with humorous materials; videos, or funny memes and anecdotes. Consider spending time with friends who are gifted at viewing every day life through a comedic lens and let yourself laugh as you appreciate and perhaps assimilate their point of view. Your sense if humor can be cultivated and enhanced. Now consider, at next opportunity, rather than walking towards the well-worn path to a Debbie Downer table, do an about face, introduce yourself to the Patti Positive group and sit right down. It may feel uncomfortable and foreign at first, but you just may leave feeling more prepared to face whatever your life challenge and you will have started a new healthy habit, "a cheerful heart."

Obedience

What Science Says

What would healthy obedience look like, for example, in a first grade classroom? We might visit a classroom, at one end of the obedience spectrum, whose students had never learned to obey, possibly as a result of their parents being overly careful not to stifle their children's freedom of choice. The classroom walls would likely be a creative muddle of crayon, markers, and paint, on the floor, play dough would be mixed with LEGO's and little Johnny would be having fun trimming little Suzy's hair. At the other end of the obedience spectrum, we might visit a class consisting of children whose parents trained them in gestapo like obedience. Not a sound would be spoken out of turn, and students would, on command, move between activities in robotic like unison, faces frozen, knowing that punishment would follow even the most minor infraction. Obviously, neither classroom scenario would be healthy or desirable for learning. Ideally, our children's classrooms consist of children who are well versed in the Golden Rule Principle. They learn respect for order and authority, and are given the opportunity and the encouragement to question, challenge, and even defy authority that violates their principles. Societal experience has demonstrated that some degree of obedience is necessary to keep order, however, "blind obedience, has proven to lead to nothing but pain and suffering."[87] (Yale University psychologist Stanley

Milgram, 1963). Obedience is healthy for the individual and for society if the decision to obey or not obey is built on sound moral principles. Examples of sound moral principles could include the Golden Rule, The Ten Commandments, the United States Constitution or the legal system. Without a well engrained base of principles upon which we, as individuals, decide to obey or to defy authority, and without sufficient fortitude to adhere to our principles, we put ourselves at risk of succumbing to the pull of social conformity, or immoral authority. Principled obedience backed by courage, though it takes much more effort to achieve, is healthy for the individual as well as for society. It is an ideal to be sought after. "Liberty is obedience to the law which one has laid down for oneself."[88] (Jean-Jacques Rousseau)

What God Says

God provided principles on which we may choose to base life decisions. The Ten Commandments were given to God's people as they entered the Promised Land, later summarized by Jesus to his followers, **"Love God. Love one Another as I have loved you."[89] (John 12:34).** Knowing these commands and adhering to them provides the moral principles upon which Christians can make decisions relative to obedience. Children are instructed to, **"Honor your father and mother so that it may be well with you, and that you may live long on the earth."[90] (Ephesians 6:1-3)** Married couples are guided in successful marriage in, **"Thou Shall not commit adultery," and "Each one**

of you also must love his wife as he loves himself, and the wife must respect her husband."[91] (Colossians 3:19) Additional commands say, **"do not steal, lie, or murder."** We are told that the way we demonstrate the love of God is through our obedience to his commands. With obedience to God, even if against immoral authority, we are given sufficient courage, **"Even though I walk through the valley of the shadow of death, I will fear no evil, for you are with me; your rod and your staff, they comfort me."[92] (Psalm 23:4)** God's instruction for living provides both the principles we need to discern moral from immoral authority and the courage we need to obey accordingly. It also promises to bring blessings. **"Blessed are those who hear the word of God and obey it."[93] (Luke 11:28)**

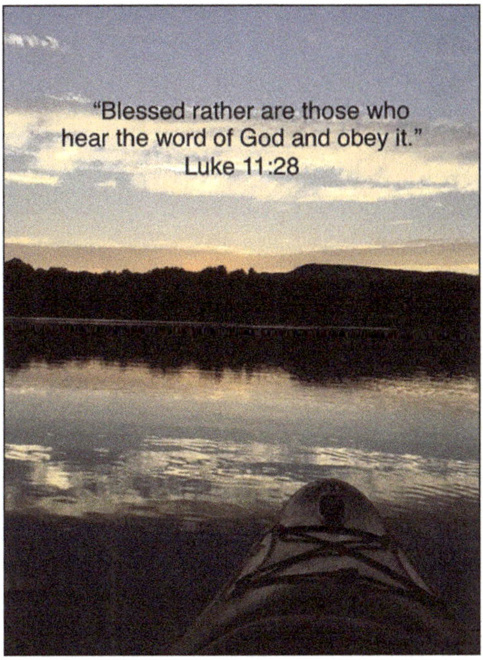

One of My Stories

I was a child of the "because I said so" parenting style of the fifties. Disobedience was met with scoldings and an occasional spanking, usually administered justly and swiftly. I carried my practice of absolute obedience to adult authority over to school, scouts and church situations. Had predators cruised the streets back then, I probably would have been a vulnerable target, even though I had been well instructed in running away from "men with offers of puppies or candy." Perceiving myself to be under the unquestioned authority of any adult, regardless of their credibility or degree of benevolence, I believed that avoidance of adult interaction was my best defense against humiliation. This, unhappily, served to curb learning opportunities and social interaction. With additional experience and education, my confidence in deciding on which principles I should base my decisions and to what authority I would choose to obey was increased. Since I have been looking to God's written Word as the source of my life principles, direction regarding obedience is much clearer to determine, and if a new question presents, I, at least, have a reliable source of reference. When courage is needed to defy worldly authority, I can ask for that too and, as promised, God delivers. **"For I am the LORD, your God, who takes hold of your right hand and says to you, Do not fear; I will help you."[94] (Isaiah 41:13)**

Write Your Story

To obey or not to obey? The next time you are called to make a decision to obey a law, a rule, or even a conventional social norm, stop and think. Does what you're about to do conform to your personal principles? If yes, feel very good about your decision to comply. If what you are asked to do violates your standards, hold firm and be true to yourself. If those around you object, you might need to call on your personal courage reserve or solicit the support of advocates. For me, God proves to be the most faithful and powerful advocate. Making decisions based on your sound moral principles and sticking to them is not only good for your own health but for the health of your children and your community. Stand strong.

Cleanliness

What Science Says

The conclusion of a cost/benefit analysis on the practice of hand washing is irrefutable. Cost of soap: pennies. Lives saved: priceless. "Effective infection prevention and control reduces health care-associated infections by at least thirty percent,"[95] according to the World Health Organization, with "just hand washing with soap alone reducing death rates from pneumonia and diarrhea by up to sixty five percent in some areas,"[96] reports Sam Stephens of the Clean the World Foundation. Medical practice was forever changed when, in 1847, Dr. Ignaz Semmelweiss, a physician in a Vienna hospital, discovered that fatal infections were spread among patients by doctors who failed to wash their hands between examinations, with some physicians going directly from handling corpses to delivering babies. Semmelweiss found that for every eleven women examined after hand washing, one fewer died. One hundred years later, Florence Nightingale promoted the case for hospital reform based on Semmelweiss's findings. Further understanding and reform followed upon the discoveries of Pasteur, Koch and Lister, ushering in the beginning of the 'Bacteriological Era. We now have powerful agencies such as Centers for Disease Control and the World Health Organization overseeing infection control and providing education. Standard infection control principles and practices include hand washing, cleaning and disinfection, waste disposal, and isolation.

What God Says

Many years before Mr. and Mrs. Semmelweiss gave birth to baby Ignaz, around 1300 B.C., the first Public Health principles were given to Moses from God. With 2.4 million people making the forty year journey from Egypt to the Promise Land, and living in crowded camp like conditions, communicable disease epidemics would have been inevitable. Cited below is a sampling of God's commands related to infection control. ***"Anyone touching a person with a "running issue" (that is, a bodily discharge), or anything upon which that person sat or lay, became "unclean". In addition, should the "toucher" touch someone without first having washed his hands, uncleanness would be transferred to the person he touched as well. Bury your waste material away from the camp."[97] (Deuteronomy 23:12–14) "Burn used dressings. Wash that contain a growth (perhaps a fungus). If the fungus/growth was removed, the garment was to be rewashed before using again. If not, it was to be burned"[98] (Leviticus 13:47–58). "If there was any doubt as to the certainty of a diagnosis of leprosy, the person was to be isolated for observation"[99] (Leviticus 13:1) "Once a person was diagnosed with a contagious condition, he was to be quarantined outside of the camp all the days wherein the plague shall be in him."[100] He was also required to wear a covering over his***

mouth, and to warn others by shouting, "Unclean, unclean!"*[101] *(Numbers 5:2–4 and Leviticus 13:45–46). In regards to unlawful lifestyles and disease, The Israelites were clearly forbidden to have any sexual relationships outside of marriage (Leviticus 18:22, 20:10–16 and Exodus 20:14). The biblical plan of husband and wife constituting an exclusive married unit (Genesis 1:27, 2:23–25; Matthew 19:3–6) certainly prevented the spread of venereal diseases, later to be the world's leading contagious diseases. Instruction was also given about keeping the water source pure, and storing food safely. God's instructions were explicit including hand washing, cleaning and disinfection, waste disposal, and isolation.

One of My Stories

After having completed another periodic infection control certification for my work as a health care provider, and while in the process of reading a few pages of the Bible every day, I was hit with a medical/spiritual revelation. "What God is telling his followers to do is consistent with current public health policy!"

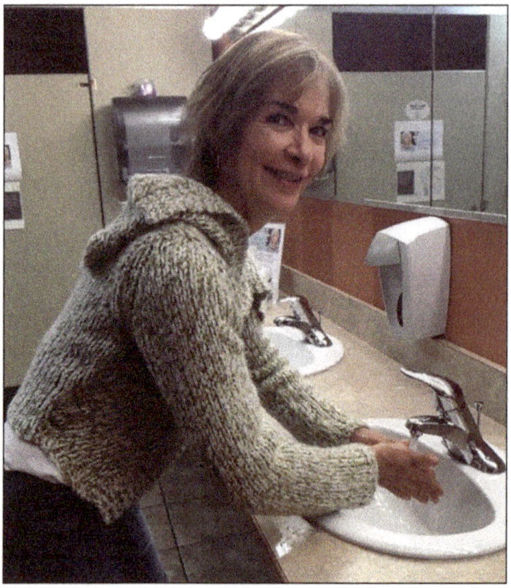

I later learned that God's public health rules were set down to prevent spreading diseases among the tightly camped Israelites enroute to Canaan. It was one of my first bible reading epiphanies that had we abided in this little bit of scripture, the subsequent deadly plagues and the HIV epidemic could have been avoided. It also hit me that germ warfare is very much akin to spiritual warfare in that in both cases the enemy is invisible and virulent, and that we are more susceptible to being harmed when our resistance is low. Needless to say, I cannot rewrite history, but I can do my small part in reducing infection by modeling some of the basic infection control practices such as hand washing and avoiding coughers and sneezers. The more powerful communicable disease risk factors such as sexual practice, drug use, and provision of clean food and water, I can be aware of and provide support as opportunity presents.

Write Your Story

Prevention is the name of the game with all disease but with infectious disease it is especially significant. Hand washing, particularly before eating, and avoiding sneezers and coughers are cost effective ways to reduce common diseases. Choosing monogamy, avoiding shared needles, and staying away from sketchy people and places are among the big guns in protecting you from the more devastating diseases. I would love to see you making important lifestyle decisions based on sound disease preventing principles rather than by what society dictates. I hope you keep in mind that, just as you cannot visualize the germ warfare you are subjected to, the spiritual warfare going on around you is also invisible and even more virulent. Wash your hands of it, friends. Choose health.

Social Support

What Science Says

YOU MAY BE AS SURPRISED AS I WAS TO learn that the connectivity and support of family and friends has as significant an impact on longevity as quitting smoking. "People who are more socially connected to family, friends, and community are happier, healthier, and live longer than people who are less well connected," several studies show. "Socially connected people live an average of 3.7 years longer than less-connected people,"[102] says study co-author Timothy B. Smith, a psychology professor at Brigham Young. A recent review of studies, on the other hand, indicates that loneliness increases mortality risk by 26%. Loneliness is identified, along with obesity and drug addiction, as a serious evolving public health problem, causation attributed partly to the dissolution and displacement of the extended family and the replacement of face to face interaction with electronic communication. To address this condition, the medical and social science communities have developed recommendations for prevention and treatment of this painful and unhealthy malady. Actively seeking new relationships through common interest clubs or activities and mending or strengthening current relationships are just two of the recommendations. "Don't think of having close relationships as a chore; think of it as part of self-care. Staying connected and involved is actually a form of taking care of yourself, just like exercise or eating right. This is an important prescription for health."[103] (Dr. Robert Waldinger, Harvard Study of Adult Development.)

What God Says

Because God created us for the purpose of loving us and for us to become a part of his family , we are, by nature, social beings. God desires not only for us to be in a loving relationship with Him but also with each other. **"And let us consider how we may spur one another on toward love and good deeds, not giving up meeting together, as some are in the habit of doing, but encouraging one another—and all the more as you see the day approaching. Above all, love each other deeply, because love covers over a multitude of sins. Offer hospitality to one another without grumbling."[104] (Hebrews 10:24-25)** Right from week one in the Garden of Eden, God created Adam and Eve for the purpose of relationship with Him and with each other. He tells us throughout the Bible to be in loving community with one another, to forgive, to be kind and to care for each other, the premiere public health prescription for health and happiness.

One of my Stories

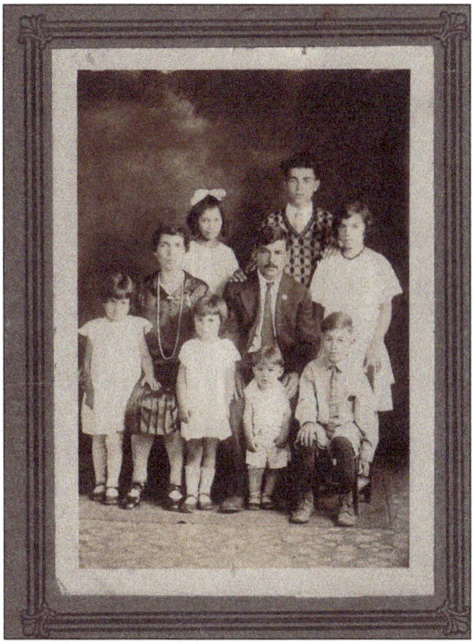

As the oldest child from a family of seven whose parents came from families of twelve and five, I never lacked for siblings, cousins, or other extended family members to establish relationships with. Holidays and birthdays were celebrated together, "come one, come all" style. Friends lived next door and across the street and we played together from after school until the fireflies lit up. We walked a mile to school together, uphill both ways I might add, and freely marched across town in group to catechism class. We saw our parents meeting at each other's homes to play cards and compare stories while we listened from our shared bedrooms. Effortlessly, we were cradled in community. If we ever felt the need for additional love and support, the hymn, "Jesus loves us, this we know because the Bible tells us so." would resonate in our heads. With the addition of marriage, motherhood, school, and job responsibilities, I failed to see the merit in expending the energy and the time required to maintain or to pursue relationships. I did enjoy the social experiences inherent in the work environment but eventually found myself wanting and lonely. Now, many years later, with much prayer and perseverance, I find myself accepting that the cost of repairing and growing current relationships and pursuing and cultivating a few healthy new ones is a wise investment of my time in terms of enjoying the rewards of good health and happiness. This means that I set aside my never ending to do list and intentionally call, text, sip coffee with, listen to music with, dance with, walk with or talk with the people God has placed in my life to be in relationship with.

Write Your Story

Even in a time when extended families are sparse and spread out, our attention is divided between devices, and our time is tight, with continual creativity, healthy relationships can be built and nurtured. Device free meals and regularly scheduled game times, bike, ski, or hike trips are a few family bonding ideas. Joining clubs, church groups or volunteering provides opportunity for starting new relationships while reaching out in humility and with forgiveness can redeem broken ones. It's a matter of making decisions to spend some of your time resource on building relationships with your long lost, soon to be, or made up with family and friends. A classic Girl Scout verse, "Make new friends. Keep the old. One is silver and the other's gold." does ring true.

Singing

What Science Says

"Sing. Sing a song. Sing out loud. Sing out strong." Research has found that singing significantly boosts our immune system by increasing the secretion of the immune protective factor, immunoglobulin A. It is increased by 150% during choral rehearsals and an incredible 240% during a choral performance. Singing also decreases our stress levels by decreasing the secretion of cortisol. One study reported a 30% reduction in cortisol levels during rehearsals and a 37% reduction during performances and, additionally, that the benefits of singing regularly seem to be cumulative. Also well documented are the physiological effects of singing on mood, confidence and mental function. It works by increasing the neurotransmitters oxytocin and the endorphins. A 1998 study found that "after anxiety/depression prone nursing-home residents took part in a singing program for a month, there were significant decreases in both anxiety and depression levels."[105](ISPS) Research has shown that "intensive singing practice can lead to long-lasting changes in both the cardiovascular and pulmonary systems. Singing is also used therapeutically in multiple neurological disorders including Parkinson's Disease."[106] (Ramig, Countryman, O'Brien, Hoehn, & Thompson, 1996). It is even effective in decreasing snoring by strengthening the muscles of the soft palate. Since singing is obviously comparable to diet and exercise in terms of health promotion and disease treatment, why then are we not belting out favorite tunes individually and in a group throughout the day? The answer is, we did once but most of stopped when we started caring about other's opinion of us. That transient discomfort can be overcome with repeated singing. We have, at our disposal, multiple ways of enjoying the health and happiness benefits of singing freely "like no one is listening." Singing in church is a wonderful way to sing and to worship at the same time. Joining a chorus or a glee club, singing at sports events, participating in karaoke, and joining young children in song are but a few opportunities. There is absolutely no limitation to singing like a rock star in the shower or in the privacy of your car or house. This is one of the few situations where "more is better." Ella Fitzgerald well knew, "the only thing better than singing, is more singing."[107]

What God Says

Jesus sang with his disciples. Moses sang with the Israelites. Apostle Paul sang in prison. King David was perpetually singing. Singing is mentioned over four hundred times in the Bible and we are given fifty direct commands to sing. It would then be safe to say, God sees singing as a very good practice and good for the welfare of his children. We are actually commanded to "**make a joyful noise to the Lord, all the earth! Serve the Lord with gladness! Come into his presence with singing!**"[108] **(Psalm 100:1-2)** We're told twice in the New Testament to sing psalms, hymns, and spiritual songs. "**Speak to one another**

in psalms, hymns, and spiritual songs, singing and making music in your hearts to the Lord."[109] (Ephesians 5:19) "Let the word of Christ dwell in you richly, teaching and exhorting one another with all wisdom, singing psalms, hymns, and spiritual songs, all with grace in your hearts to God."[110] (Colossians 3:16) Anything Jesus models or God commands is meant for our health and welfare. With a Bible that is infused with singing, both worshipful and celebratory, there can be no doubt that singing is indeed what researchers are beginning to discover, "like an infusion of the perfect tranquilizer, the kind that both soothes your nerves and elevates your spirits."

One of My Stories

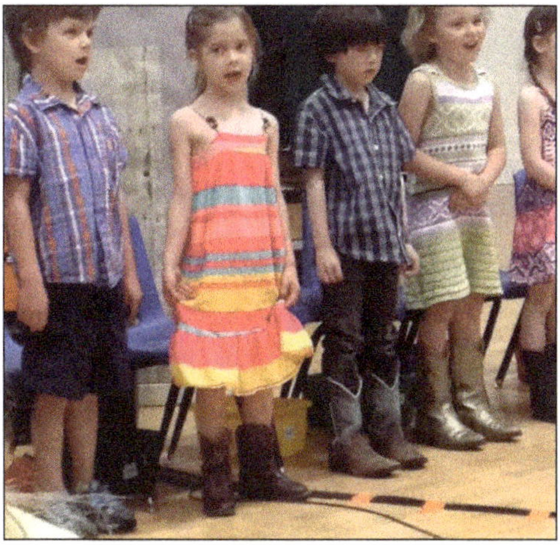

I loved singing lullabies to my infant children as I rocked them to sleep. As soon as they learned to talk, however, whenever I broke into song, they would sweetly say, "you're such a good dancer, Mommy. Why don't you dance instead?" So I was not Aretha Franklin. My singing career evolved from singing alone in the car or house to singing with others at church. I will now pretty much join in any singing situation, be it a hockey game or my grand kids school concert. If my mood needs a boost, cranking up "golden oldies" in the car and singing along never fails to pick me up. What never ceases to amaze me is the beautiful harmony emitted by any mix of choral singers, whether it is trained professionals, a church choir or a mix of first and second graders. I have witnessed the uplifting effects of singing in various venues be it rock concerts, nursing homes or nursery schools. I see singing as one of the many God given gifts that is encouraged to enjoy as often as possible for health and for happiness.

Write Your Story

Singing makes you healthier, happier, and more approachable. It can calm and it can excite. It improves snoring, stuttering, memory, and enhances pulmonary and cardiovascular function. It is fun, free, and can be done anywhere without the need for expensive equipment. It will not cook dinner nor will it do the dishes but it is otherwise difficult to deny it's virtue and it's utility. Singing is too great a gift to let your concern over other's opinion of your virtuosity keep you from enjoying its pleasure and its benefits. Sing in the shower, sing in car, sing when you're walking. Sing where you are. Sing by yourself or join a group. Consider a choir or a professional troupe. If you praise God with song, like I do, the benefits can soar right out of this world. It is said by those who sing for their supper that "singing daily for at least ten minutes, reduces your stress, clears your sinuses, improves your posture, and can even help you live longer." Be like Fred Allen. He loved singing so much that even though "The first time he sang in the church choir; two hundred people changed their religion, he continued to sing."[111] (Fred Allen)

Love

What Science Says

"Love doesn't make the world go round but it is what makes the ride worthwhile."[112] (Franklin P. Jones, reporter and humorist). Merriam-Webster defines love as "a feeling of strong or constant affection for a person: attraction that includes sexual desire : the strong affection felt by people who have a romantic relationship. : a person you love in a romantic way."[113] I prefer C.S. Lewis description of love as "not an affectionate feeling, but a steady wish for the loved person's ultimate good as far as it can be obtained."[114] Repeated studies, using married men and women as subjects, have been conducted on the effects of love on health. Results overwhelmingly suggest that love is indeed very good for each partner's health with "married people living longer, have better access to health care, enjoying a more satisfying sex life, experiencing less stress, living a healthier lifestyle, and having lower rates of heart disease, diabetes, and depression compared to their single counterparts." The list of health perks conferred by marriage is so long, in fact, that the U.S. Department of Health and Human Services has made it a centerpiece of its two-year-old, $5 million national media campaign to promote wedded bliss.

What God Says

Christianity does not direct us to focus on finding the right person; it calls us to "become the right person." Christian marriage authority, Gary Thomas, goes so far as to challenge the world's perspective on the purpose of marriage; "What if God designed marriage to make us holy more than to make us happy?"[115] **"God demonstrates his perfect love for us, his children, in not basing his love for us on our merit."[116] (Deuteronomy 7:7-8; Romans 5:7-8).** The most infamous recitation on love, spoken at many weddings, was recorded by Apostle Paul, **"Love is patient, love is kind. It does not envy, it does not boast, it is not proud. It does not dishonor others, it is not self-seeking, it is not easily angered, it keeps no record of wrongs."[117] (1 Corinthians 13:4-5). "God alone is the source of love."[118] (1 John 4:7-8); he "poured out his love into our hearts by the Holy Spirit, whom he has given us."[119] (Romans 5:5)**. God's love then awakens a response in those who accept it. God designed and gifted us marriage as a way to become better people by loving our spouses unconditionally. **"He who finds a wife [or she who finds a husband] finds a good thing, and obtains favor from the Lord."[120] (Proverbs 18:22)** Committed partners gain both happiness and health in encouraging each other's spiritual, physical and emotional growth.

One of My Stories

I am married now for the fifth time. I can either be perceived as the person least likely to author a "Dear Abbey" romance advise column or as a person with the wisdom that comes with having learned from multiple poor marital decisions. The difference between my current marriage and my past marriages is that both my husband Fred and myself, though each on our own individual spiritual path, have said yes to the promptings of God, both committed to doing God's will for our lives. The three of us are now in a marriage that was well worth the wait, God, Fred and me. From a worldly perspective, it seems paradoxical that the less I look to Fred for happiness, but instead strive to become more like Jesus, the happier I become. I keep in mind who my Heavenly Father-in-law is and view Fred through his eyes. God's instructions are clear; **"Each husband must love his wife as he loves himself, and the wife must respect her husband."[121] (Ephesians 5:33)** This is contrary to the world's instruction, but then the world's instruction has never served me well. Our marriage continues to be challenged by whatever the world throws our way but, as long as we put God first in our lives, and live

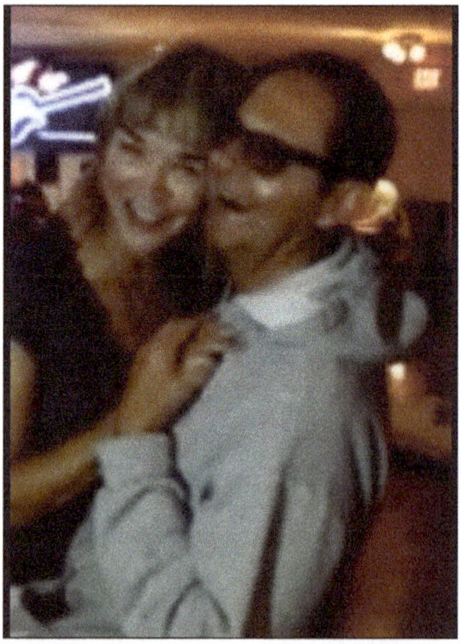

according to his rules, not ours, we continue to enjoy a marriage designed in heaven.

Write Your Story

It has been established that love through marriage is excellent for our health. It is also, sadly, well known that fifty percent of first marriages end in divorce, worse with remarriages. Interestingly, statistics also reveal that couples who pray together, stay together ninety nine percent of the time. How might you glean from this information to increase your chance of finding yourself in a committed healthy marriage? If you are unmarried, beware of the world's dictum to allow "feelings" to reign over your decisions. Feelings are fickle and misleading, seducing us to make regrettable choices every time. If you are already in a marriage, you might consider viewing the act of "praying" as an effective action of love and imitate or simulate it. Why not consider practicing other love actions toward your spouse such as forgiving, respecting, listening, and comforting to name a few. If your spouse is seemingly unappreciative, do it anyway. Do not let pride, the biggest handicapper, get in your way. You're a winner either way. At the very least, you grow as a person. At best, you grow as a couple. You will learn that loving unconditionally is its own reward.

Water

What Science Says

We can go about three weeks without food, whereas we can only go about three to four days without water before utter dehydration and death. With up to sixty percent of the human adult body composed of water, it is essential in regulating body temperature, moistening tissues in the eyes, nose and mouth, protecting body organs and tissues, carrying nutrients and oxygen to cells, lubricating joints, and flushing out waste products. It also helps dissolve minerals and nutrients to make them accessible to our body. Water is a freely flowing, effective and safe weight loss tool, a side effect free, late afternoon energy booster, and a cost effective beauty aid, plumping the skin and reducing wrinkles. According to Mayo Clinic, "women require 11.5 cups of water per day, men 15.5 cups, of which twenty percent will typically come from food."[122] The amount of water required will vary with exercise and environment. More is not always better and, in very large quantities, in fact, water can be hazardous to our health. Regarding sports drinks, "if we're working out for less than an hour, water will do just fine. We do not deplete electrolyte and glycogen reserves until we have been exercising intensely for over an hour,"[123] according to Dr. Stanley Goldfarb, professor of medicine at the University of Pennsylvania. The best hydrating beverage is not blue, pink, bubbled, fizzled, beautifully bottled or budget breaking. It is clear, clean, colorless, free costing, right out of the faucet water. In this case, "too good to be true" is true. We may drink to that.

What God Says

We only need to go six verses into the Bible to read about water. It then is found streaming through the Bible at least 722 more times. God said, **"Let there be an expanse in the midst of the waters and let it separate water from water. So God made the expanse and separated the water under the expanse from the water above it."[124] (Genesis 1:6-8)** Water was one of the two get well items God's angel ministered to the prophet Elijah when Elijah was at the end of his rope, worn out and depressed. **"All of a sudden, an angelic messenger touched him and said, "Get up and eat." Elijah looked and right there by his head was a cake baking on hot coals and a jug of water. He ate and drank and then slept some more."[125] (1Kings19:4-5)** The twenty third psalm includes water as part of a visual retreat for anyone who is in need of comfort, **"He takes me to lush pastures, he leads me to refreshing water."[126] (Psalm**

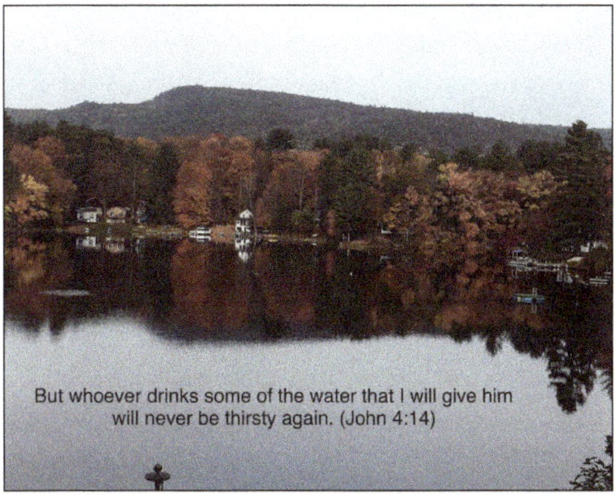

23:2) Water is a gift offering in **(Matthew 10:42) "And whoever gives only a cup of cold water to one of these little ones in the name of a disciple, I tell you the truth, he will never lose his reward."**[127] Multiple times the Holy Spirit is symbolically referred to as **"living water,"** supporting the life giving quality of water

One of My Stories

While growing up, the cost of water nicely matched the family's budget line allotted for beverages, provincially protecting me from developing a taste for sugary drinks. I remain loyal to out of the faucet water to quench my thirst, sometimes kicking it up a notch with a slice of lime or a bubble or two. To trick myself into meeting my recommended daily water quota, I keep a lovely looking container of water in the car or at my desk, and also sip cups of hot water to keep myself warm in the summer air conditioning while simultaneously hydrating. I sadly marvel at the effectiveness of marketing in selling bottled water with "revenues for the U.S. bottled water market in 2016 at nearly sixteen billion in wholesale dollars". While expensive bottled water does not contribute any more to good health than free tap water, it does, however, contribute significantly to global warming and to pollution. I turn on the faucet and drink to health, mine and the planet's. While sometimes slowing down enough to savor a glass of water, I am mindful of both the physical and the spiritual sustenance I am receiving through my drinking of both the liquid and the "living" water.

Write Your Story

You can choose to view water as the essential life source it is. It is yours to tap into and it's free; your multipurpose magic potent. Start with eight cups a day just to keep your body working. Need weight loss? Have a glass of liquid belly filler before each meal. Afternoon slump got you down? Treat or prevent that slump with a glass of the cool wet stuff. How about a quick cure for work out poop out? Don't forget to bring along your reusable bottle of lemon flavored water to lube those muscles and pump up your circulation. Need to cool down after your work out? If you've got a pool of it, jump in. If not, spritz it on your face or pour it right over your head. You've got the idea. It's one of the best health values money does not need to buy. As you continue to revel in the wonders of wonderful water, you might consider it's Creator, and develop a thirst for "Living" Water.

REPENTANCE

What Science Says

REPENTANCE IS BIG. THE WEBSTER Dictionary defines repentance as "the turning from sin or wrong doing and the changing of one's mind."[128] In the medical realm, the confession aspect of repentance is recognized for its therapeutic value. Research shows that "no matter how we start, the act of sharing out loud our struggles, our behaviors, our fears, our problems or joys, the benefits of confessing who we are to another human being can be freeing, strengthening and releasing."[129] (Dr. Thomas, licensed psychologist, author, International University of Professional Studies) Alcoholics Anonymous, founded in 1935, often described as "God given," has demonstrated consistent success in providing a path to recovery for the heretofore incurable alcoholic. The twelve steps of AA is a detailed approach to repentance. It starts with the admission of powerlessness over the alcoholic's current life, followed by the turning of his will and his life over to a "higher power" (God). The next steps involve "making a searching and fearless moral inventory of himself, admitting to God, himself, and to another human being the exact nature of his wrongs, becoming entirely ready to be changed, and humbly asking God to remove his defects of character."[130] The process culminates in a spiritual awakening into a new life as a sober, healthy person. This recovering individual continues to take a personal inventory and, when wrong, promptly admits it. As a result of this change in thinking, the transformed person emerges a healthier, happier version of himself with a desire to help others to do the same. This desire to help others serves to maintain and to promote further growth. The AA twelve step program has been used as a model for multiple subsequent programs designed to help people overcome addictions or other harmful strongholds on their lives. There are no short cuts to the change process but, if one is willing to do the work, the results are monumentally life changing for the individual and for everyone whose lives they touch.

What God Says

"Repent: for the kingdom of heaven is at hand."[131] (Matthew 4:17), was declared by Jesus at the onset of his ministry. To better understand the message, we need to know the context from which it was given. In Jesus' time, many people were discontent under the burden of Jewish religious law and Roman rule. Jesus offered them hope by inviting them to go in a new direction, to repent from their sins and to adopt a new way of thinking; a change of heart. **"For whatever is in your heart determines what you say."[132] (Matthew 12:34)** It also determines behavior. God offers healing through repentance to us individually or to our nation as a whole. **"If my people, who are called by my name, will humble themselves and pray and seek my face and turn from their wicked ways, then I will hear from heaven, and I will forgive their sin and will heal their land."[133] (2 Chronicles 7:14)** To assure continued growth towards being more Christ like, Christians are directed to continue the process of confession, repentance and turning direction. A favorite prayer to this end is, "**Search me, O God, and know my heart: try me, and know my thoughts. See if there be any wicked way in me, and lead me in the way everlasting."[134] (Psalm 139:23-24)** With every opportunity to recognize an undesirable thought or behavior, to confess it, to repent, and to change our hearts, we become more like Christ.

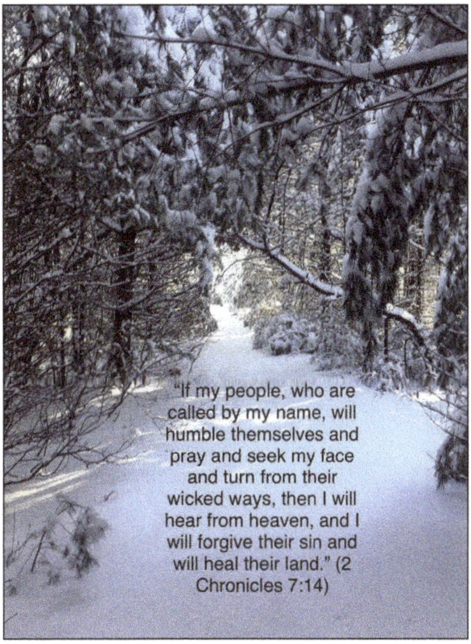

One of My Stories

How could I repent when I never did anything wrong? For every decision I made, I could point to societal mores for which my choices were perfectly acceptable, if not applauded. There did, however, come a point of extreme discomfort when there was not another relationship, new home, college degree, job change, fitness technique, or mood altering substance that could fill the gaping hole in my soul. Having reached the end of myself and in complete desperation, my knees hit the floor and I prayed. The Holy Spirit planted a desire in my heart for radical change and caused me to recognize the error of my ways. Opportunity was presented to confess and to repent, resulting in some changed behaviors and a thirst for truth. The process was frustratingly slow until I was exposed to, what I knew in my heart to be the truth, the Bible. Though my life may now appear simple by world standards, as a "reborn" me, I joyfully know the truth; that life is about love of God and love of others. I experience joy and genuine freedom in choosing to go where God leads me.

Write Your Story

If you experience anything from a mild to a profound unrest whenever you find yourself without a source of external stimulation, know that this could just be all the incentive you need to halt, do an about face, and to march off to a more joyous and free future. If you have a relationship with God or even if a small part of you considers that there could be something, somewhere more powerful than you, this would be a great time to invite in a little help. Even a, "God, please help," will suffice. The rest of the repentance process; acknowledging your transgressions, asking God for forgiveness, and turning towards new thinking and new behavior may be done several ways. You will need some source of help and guidance. You could join a Twelve Step Program, enlist the help of a counselor or pastor and/or join a bible based church with a solid bible study program, as a few suggestions. I will not even allude to a time schedule because it is so variable. I can overwhelmingly attest to the value of making this fresh start. It is well worth the time and the effort it takes to turn your life around through repentance. I can affirm that what God promised me has come to pass. " **Repent, then, and turn to God, so that your sins may be wiped out, that times of refreshing may come from the Lord."[135] (Acts 3:19)**

Sports

What Science Says

Game on! Sports can help us reach our fitness goals and maintain a healthy weight. Sports participation can also encourage healthy decision-making such as not smoking and not drinking. Breast cancer and osteoporosis risk is also reduced. Learning that hard work, through sport participation, pays off in achieving goals, develops perseverance and self-confidence. Participants can also become a part of a supportive social network, developing friendships and being given social and even business opportunities. Whether the sporting event is lost or won, every participant is a winner. Being a star athlete does, however, carry with it, not only opportunity, but also responsibility. Nick Foles, NFL quarterback, modeled both integrity and humility in leading his team to win the 2018 Super Bowl, "Just like when I hoisted the Lombardi Trophy, the reason I smiled, was that, in that moment, I realized I didn't need that trophy to define who I was because I was already in Christ."[136] (Nick Foles). Some "super" athletes, sadly, sit on the other end of the integrity spectrum. While budding young athletes are watching, they irresponsibly model violence, egotism, and disrespect. Like it or not, as well spoken by Winston Churchill, "Responsibility is the price of greatness."[137]

What God Says

The Bible repeatedly uses athletics analogously to demonstrate various virtues. Apostle Paul uses athletics to expound on the merits of integrity in the book of 2 Timothy, "**If anyone competes in athletics, he is not crowned unless he competes according to the rules.**"[138] **(2 Timothy 2:5)** Discipline is described in the book of Corinthians, comparing a transient earthly crown to an everlasting heavenly crown. **"Everyone who competes in the games goes into strict training. They do it to get a crown that will not last, but we do it to get a crown that will last forever."**[139] **(Corinthians 9:25) "And let us run with perseverance the race marked out for us."**[140] **(Hebrews 12:1)** Scripture compares the value of perseverance in athletics with perseverance in one's spiritual journey. Though the Bible does not specifically advocate sports participation, particular scripture is consistent with success in sports as well as success in life; maintenance of a healthy body, discipline, and perseverance.

One of My Stories

My sister Mary takes first place in having used sports to help bring her through a devastating life situation. Sport participation was not new to my sister. She had had a very positive and strong sports history. During high school, Mary enjoyed encouraging her team to victory as a most effervescent cheerleader. Go Bulldogs! She ran circles around the track team and also developed an interest in tennis. In addition to the spiritual, family and friend support Mary was provided, she found sports participation to help her in multiple other ways. It was competitive tennis that she was drawn to when she needed something more to relieve stress and help rebuild her self-esteem. Through playing tennis regularly, she was able to keep in great shape, make good and supportive friends, network, and, more importantly, feel successful again. My niece, Grace, has benefited from observing her mom's perseverance and discipline and by carrying these qualities over to her own life, cause her to be on her way to becoming an accomplished dancer. Mary's son Chris demonstrates these same winning strategies in his music pursuits. As a family, they are on top of their game with the benefits of sports participation continuing to provide a positive force.

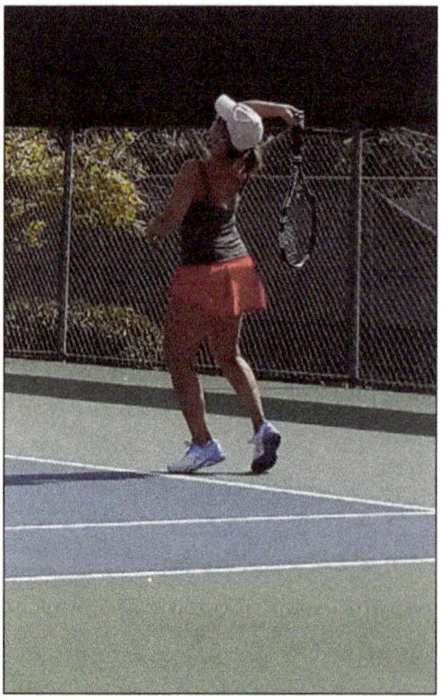

Write Your Story

Maybe you do not consider yourself a Michael Jordan or a Serena Williams but it is not necessary for you to be anywhere near that skill level to benefit from sports participation. Even if you do have a sports history but find you are now more inclined to enjoy sweating vicariously through spectatorship, this could be your call to action. It may be just the time to resurrect your old tennis racket or baseball glove. Alternately, you could be ready to learn a new skill to better match your current ability level. There are several new games options including pickleball, ultimate frisbee, or foosball to choose from. Whether your involvement is physically challenging and highly competitive, cheering enthusiastically from the sidelines, or somewhere in between, sports can enhance your physical and emotional health. It can also build your skills in perseverance and discipline while providing social opportunity. Do keep in mind that you are being observed and you will be emulated. You might even practice these responses such as these ahead of time; "gosh, did I really miss that ball and lose the championship for the team?" or "Yay for that quarter back. He sure ran fast. Such a shame he tripped on a pigeon in the end zone." So it's one, two, three, four. Join a team and you will score.

Encouragement

What Science Says

Sometimes referred to as "verbal sunshine," encouragement is one of the most powerful ways to build a child, build an adult, or build an entire company to reach their full potential. It is the most cost effective way to influence successful thinking, while improving the health and the welfare of the encourager as well as the encouraged. In Ken Blanchard's best-selling book, The One Minute Manager, Blanchard's number one key to building a successful company is to "Catch somcone doing something good and praise them for one minute."[141] Ralph Carol Dweck, Ph.D., a researcher at Stanford University, takes the art of encouragement to the next level, observing that "The critical difference between praise and encouragement, is that encouragement breaks down barriers and unlocks potential while praise can create ceilings."[142] It has been proven that if someone who achieves an A on a test, for instance, is praised for their "smartness," they will generally protect this desired label by being cautious, whereas if someone who receives an A is praised for their "hard work," they will be encouraged to work even harder thereby becoming more successful." A commonly used "at a boy" type praise does indeed show someone that we noticed them for doing a commendable act but a higher octane encouragement can be provided if we make the effort to know what motivates the person we are encouraging, while appreciating them just as they are. We have then set the stage to encourage them for their successful efforts and perseverance. We may then witness the glow and the enhanced growth that this focused encouragement can provide.

What God Says

Proverbs 18:21 says, **"The tongue has the power of life and death."** God, our Creator, is clear in directing us to help each other to grow through encouragement. **"Therefore encourage one another and build each other up, just as, in fact, you are doing."**[143] Encouragement is a gift, like kindness, that the more you give away, the more you receive. **"If you give, you will receive. Your gift will return to you in full measure, pressed down, shaken together to make room for more, and running over. Whatever measure you use in giving—large or small—it will be used to measure what is given back to you."**[144] **(Luke 6:38)** The second of the two great commands God gives us in order for us to live the best possible life on earth and in heaven is to **"love one another as He loves us."** The act of encouragement is a mutually beneficial way to accomplish this.

One of My Stories

"My teacher thought I was smarter than I was-so I was."[145] (Written by a 6 year old.) Out of the mouths of babes comes some of the most profound and succinct perspectives on life. Teachers, as well as parents, are in unique positions to alter the course of young lives with a few choice words. My heart has

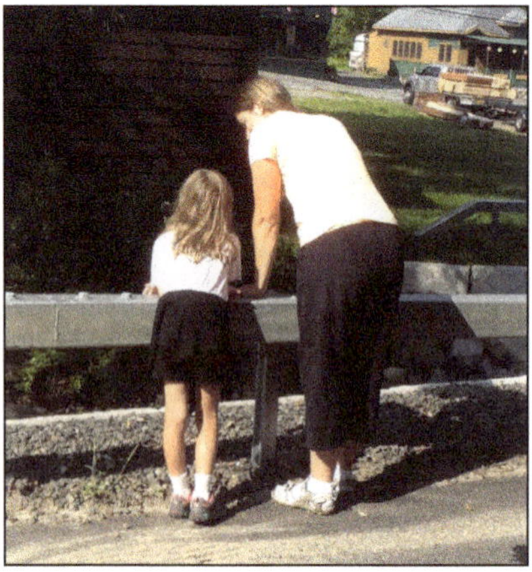

been broken with stories of the crushing effects of a few discouraging words from a significant adult to a young child. I am happy to say I do not have to look very far to observe the reverse scenario. I often have the privilege of personally witnessing the effects of my daughter Angela's going to any length to encourage her children through her words and her actions. She attentively and reflectively listens, not only when it's convenient, but whenever her finely tuned mama receptors perceive a need. I marvel at seeing her enthusiastically get up at the crack of dawn to travel for hours to provide a fun growth opportunity for her children, then stay up, sometimes until the early morning hours, to complete her own professional

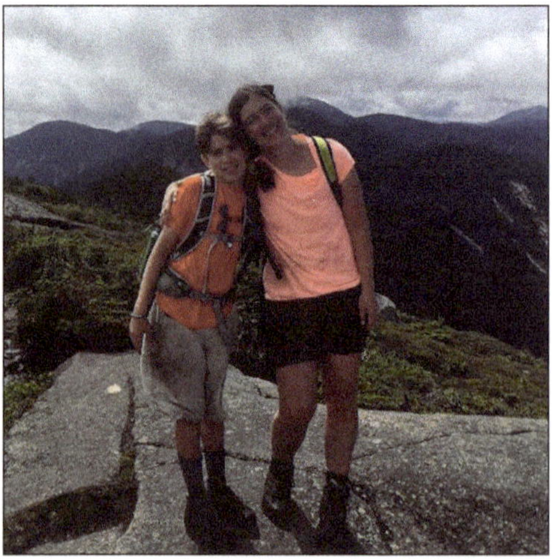

responsibilities. It melts my heart to see the positive effects of her and her husband's encouragement on their children, my grandchildren. I reflect on how the world would be changed if this encouraging approach became more universal.

Write Your Story

What makes you feel encouraged? Do you feel more encouraged after being interviewed by a potential employer who smiles at you during an interview or one who scowls? You have everything it takes to be a vessel of encouragement as you sail through your day. In you is the power to illuminate sales clerks, passersby, friends, and family. Be careful to guard your smile as you sail along, not allowing it to droop in the wind. It is a wonderful way for you to light up your piece of the world. You may even want to consider offering up an entire day to watch very closely for opportunity to encourage anyone fortunate enough to be in your path. Give a smile and a hello, a hand on a shoulder, a sincere thank you, a sharing of a helpful personal story, or a praise for great effort. Stand beside or sit next to. At the end of the day, rerun your experiences in your mind. On day two, you may decide to repeat day one. Be aware, however, friends and family are watching. You may be imitated and soon find that your little piece of the world is becoming a bit happier, healthier and more aglow with verbal sunshine.

Rest

What Science Says

"For me, not working is the real work."[146] (Stephen King). Taking time off to rest is difficult for many Americans, proven by our track record of taking off about one half of the days as our European counterparts even though time off is well demonstrated to increase lifespan. "Men who take a vacation every year reduce their overall risk of death by about twenty percent and specifically their risk of death from heart disease by up to thirty percent."[147] (Framingham Study) Research has also found that "women who don't take time off are more likely to suffer from depression and, according to one study, are fifty percent more likely to have a heart attack." "Vacation takers also have fewer stress-related physical complaints such as headaches, backaches, and heart irregularities."[148] (study from the University of Vienna) additionally, "workers who use their vacation days are more likely to be promoted than those who forfeit them."[149] (Project "Time Off") It turns out that any length "vacation" is health promoting. Napping, for instance, offers various benefits for healthy adults, including relaxation, reduced fatigue, increased alertness, improved mood, and improved performance and memory; a sixty minute nap proving to be the ideal length for memory improvement."[150] (Mayo Clinic) Research also suggests that, "When faced with long tasks such as studying before a final exam or doing your taxes, it is best to impose brief breaks on yourself. Brief mental breaks will actually help you stay focused on your task." (Alejandro Lleras, University of Illinois) Lleras's study recommends a simple exercise called 20-20-20. His study findings recommend that "every twenty minutes or so, stare at something at least twenty feet away from you for at least twenty seconds. This simple exercise will help rest your eyes and prevent fatigue, neck and back soreness, headaches, and blurred vision."[151] A practice called "waking rest" is associated with memory-related brain activity during quiet rest and suggests that in our daily lives, moments of unoccupied rest may serve an essential cognitive function, contributing to memory consolidation. "Waking rest can last from five to twenty minutes once or multiple times per day, and should take place in an area where the participant feels safe, comfortable, and can remain uninterrupted by outside influences. It should involve a low-energy or repetitive activity that does not require focused thought to perform (e.g. yard work, folding laundry, or walking the dog.)" Work to live happy and healthy, not to work yourself into an early grave. Vacation, naps and waking rest, are essentials for your health. It's a bonus that "waking rest" activities are usually very pleasurable.

What God Says

How important rest is to our health and well-being is made clear by God placing the command to rest in the second book of the Bible and as number three of the Ten Commandments. **"Remember the Sabbath day**

by keeping it holy. Six days you shall labor and do all your work, but the seventh day is a Sabbath to the LORD your God. On it you shall not do any work, neither you, nor your son or daughter, nor your male or female servant, nor your animals, nor any foreigner residing in your towns."[152] (Exodus 20:8-19) God, our loving Father, also invites us to call on him whenever we are in need of rest, be it physical or emotional **"Come unto me, all ye that labour and are heavy laden, and I will give you rest. Take my yoke upon you, and learn of me; for I am meek and lowly in heart: and ye shall find rest unto your souls. For my yoke is easy, and my burden is light."[153] (Matthew 11:28-30)** Those of us who call God Lord, may look forward to both worldly and eternal rest. **"The Lord is my shepherd; I shall not want. He makes me to lie down in green pastures: he leads me beside the still waters. He restores my soul: he leads me in the paths of righteousness for his name's sake."[154] (Psalm 23:1-5)**

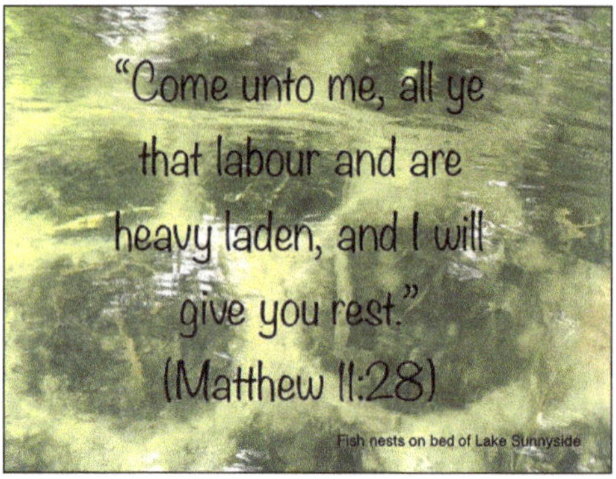

Fish nests on bed of Lake Sunnyside

One of My Stories

The closest I came to rest, aside from sleep, in my formative years was day dreaming. This restful escape served me well in nurturing my, now very utilitarian, creative and problem solving skills. I later learned the fine art of napping, passed down to me by generations of skilled practitioners. I have incorporated the science of the nap and have fine-tuned this skill in terms of timing, duration, environmental factors and other contributing variables. "Waking rest," though I did not previously know it by name, is an additional skill I lay claim to by, taking breaks from the task of writing or reading to pull weeds, dust furniture, or scan my cabin for decorating possibilities. I have ultimately learned to enjoy premium grade rest, the kind that is possible even through simultaneously running pandemics and civil unrest, only recently, through development of a closer relationship with God. That relationship has followed a sequence of steps; acceptance, obedience, faith and, most recently, trust. God does, as He promises, **"restores my soul: and he leads me in the paths of righteousness for his name's sake." (Psalm 23:1-5)**

Write Your Story

You are exhausted. You routinely sleep seven hours a night and are just too tired to exercise after work. Besides, you have dinner to prepare, children's homework to review and some catch-up communication with a spouse for a bit in the evening. There is no time to fit in rest; or is there? You are well aware of the benefits of rest for your health and that of your family so you are ready to make a few changes. Let us develop a template that allows for flexibility depending on the nature and the pace of your job responsibilities. You might start the day by arising a few minutes early and put together a crock pot dinner. Arrive to work early enough to greet everyone with a smile and have time to savor the aroma and taste of a cup of coffee or the equivalent there of. Perform your duties, no matter what they are, with enthusiasm. At your scheduled, or first available, break, move yourself out of the work situation as well as you can, recognizing that the move may be only in your mind in some cases. Move around, change the view and the subject as much as possible. At lunch, eat lightly then possibly walk with an upbeat friend. During the afternoon break, go to a quieter room, drink a glass of water, take a deep breath, sit back and close your eyes or leaf through an appealing magazine. After work, depending on the maturity of your children, have them either set the table or sit and watch a fun show with them cuddled on the couch with your feet up. At catch-up time with your spouse, plan your next regularly scheduled vacation with the same commitment that you would give to scheduling your children's medical care. This may sound like a lot of extra effort but you do know that any good change takes effort and adjustment at the onset. Not only will you be healthier and happier but you will be modeling a healthier and happier lifestyle for those you love.

Forgiveness

What Science Says

SIMPLY PUT, FORGIVENESS IS LETTING GO of grudges and bitterness. It is an action to be taken, not just a feeling that happens. Forgiveness is about healing yourself with no participation of the perpetrator necessary. Resentment, on the other hand, is a bitter indignation at having been treated unfairly. Resentment is the product of unforgiveness. Studies have found that the act of forgiveness can reap huge rewards for your health, lowering your risk of heart attack; improving cholesterol levels and sleep; and reducing pain, blood pressure, and levels of anxiety, depression and stress. Additionally, research points to an increase in the forgiveness-health connection as you age. Alcohol addiction is an example of the powerful detrimental effects of resentment. The Big Book of Alcoholics Anonymous, declares, "Resentment destroys more alcoholics than anything else."[155] Members are instructed to "show the offender the same tolerance, pity, and patience that he would cheerfully grant a sick friend." and further, to ask himself, "How can I be helpful to him", and adding "God save me from being angry."[156] Learning the process of overcoming resentment literally saves the lives of people who are afflicted with the disease of alcoholism, a powerful testimony to the healing power of forgiveness.

What God Says

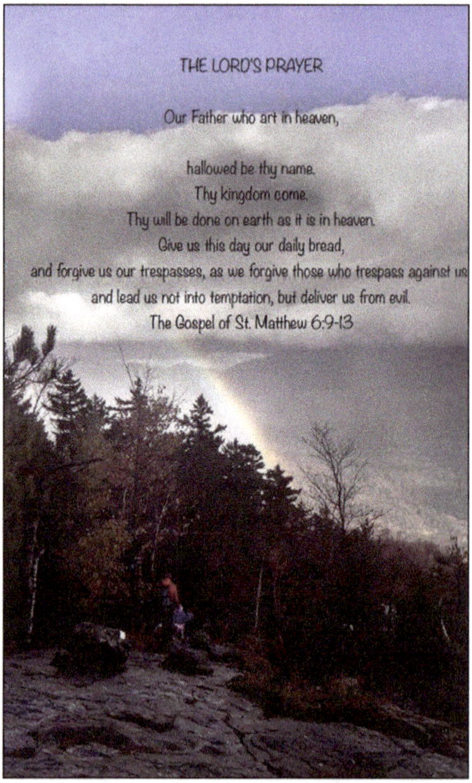

The most effective "how to" on forgiveness is found in the Bible. Biblical forgiveness is, first of all, a decision to release the offender from the guilt of his sin. We then refuse to bring up the offense to use against him. We refuse to think about the offense or to talk to others about the offense. If possible, we reconcile with the offender. Jesus stand on forgiveness is decisive, instructing his disciples to forgive **"70 times seven times"[157] in the Gospel of (Matthew 18:21-22).** In both the gospel of Matthew and the gospel of Luke, Jesus includes a reciprocal formula in the Lord's Prayer, **"Forgive us as we forgive others."[158] (Matthew 6:12; Luke 11:4)**

One of My Stories

After making a financially imprudent divorce agreement with an abusive husband and later finding he had also been unfaithful, I was faced with a decision; take the high road of forgiveness or wallow in a well justified resentment. My automatic default would have been regret and anger, resulting in making myself very ill. In this case, I made a decision to forgive. I prayed for him and put my focus on living in the present and planning for the future. I memorized and practiced Apostle Paul's instruction to the early church, **"Finally, brothers and sisters, whatever is true, whatever is noble, whatever is right, whatever is pure, whatever is lovely, whatever is admirable—if anything is excellent or praiseworthy—think about such things."[159] (Philippians 4:8).** I was eventually able to see my ex as an imperfect person, like me, with perhaps a different variety and scheduling of transgressions. As a bonus, I was delighted to find that forgiving him his offense, helped me to forgive myself for my mistakes. Once again, when I followed God's written Word to confess my sins and turn away from doing them again, I experienced a peace and a freedom second to none.

Write Your Story

Suppose your coworker had spread a false rumor that prevented you from getting a promotion. Your boss found out the truth but the promotion had been already given to someone else. No one would criticize you for denouncing your conspirer or for letting the entire office know what they did. What if, instead, you stopped, took a deep breath and made a decision to forgive them? What if you made the decision even if you did not feel like it? Instead of your energy and time being diverted to anger and resentment, it would be used to lift your self esteem, nourish your relationships, and grow your character. Sometimes a battle is lost but the war is won.

Music

What Science Says

Albert Einstein declared, "If I were not a physicist, I would probably be a musician."[160] We can only speculate on his reasoning but I'm thinking that the scientific side of Einstein was aware of the proven health benefits of music while the personal side of Albert just wanted to get a groove on. McGill University in Montreal studied 400 research papers regarding the neurochemistry of music, and found many benefits including a boosted immune system. The findings from the university concluded that "music increases levels of immunoglobulin A that helps your body fend off viruses. It also boosts antibodies responsible for destroying bacteria that slips past your body's security systems."[161] Valorie Salimpoor, a neuroscientist at McGill University, injected eight music-lovers with a radioactive substance that binds to dopamine receptors after they listened to their favorite music. A PET scan showed that large amounts of dopamine were released, which biologically caused the participants to feel emotions like happiness, excitement, and joy. Depending on the genre, tempo, lyrics, and intensity, music can motivate to exercise, lower blood pressure through relaxation, lull to sleep, and create an array of emotions. Supported by these, and other findings, music therapy is used as an effective milieu in treating chronic disease, pain, and mood disorders.

What God Says

Once upon a time, 2009 BC to be more precise, King Saul's court was at their wits end trying to find something or someone to quell the king's emotional distress. A servant remembered young David, the shepherd boy, renowned for his harp playing skills. David's music, so it is written, was the only effective method for calming King Saul. David's later military victories were also celebrated in song in 1 Samuel 18:6–7. The Bible is virtually bursting at the seams with music. We are commanded to communicate with each other **"with psalms, hymns, and songs from the Spirit. Sing and make music from your heart to the Lord"**[162] **(Ephesians 5:19)** Through psalms and hymns, music comprises entire books of the Bible. Even before the beginning of our time on earth, the angels were created with musical abilities and sang at the creation of the earth (see Ezekiel 28:13-14) We continue to glorify God with music every chance we can. As intended, music worships God while nourishing and healing our bodies and our souls

One of My Stories

If this "Sue" walks or runs to the sound of "Run Around Sue", instead of to the sound of street traffic, my running time is much better and my energy level soars. Singing "Amazing Grace" with Anne Murray or "Dancing Queen" with ABBA, while driving, lifts my spirits within minutes. It is sometimes awkward, however, to satisfy the urge to pull over and twirl a few twirls or shake a quick hip. At home, my energy level can go from zero to seventy if I allow my husband's drum practicing to lift me from couch sitting to whirling and twirling around the living room. Music is not only fun and motivating but has proven to be very therapeutic. I've very recently personally witnessed a stunning example of the effectiveness of music therapy. My ninety-two year old mom was moved from a firm stance of resistance to a spirit of willing cooperation with her physical therapist through my daughter Angela's playing of her Nana's favorite music. It was amazing to watch my mom's eyebrows raise and her eyes sparkle as she took steps forward to Glenn Miller's "In the Mood". Prior to this, my granddaughter, Schuyler, had relaxed "Nana" in ICU by quietly strumming her guitar while singing her a love song. The mood altering and healing effects of music are profound and pervasive. Our appreciation for music, to me, is one of the special gifts God has instilled within us. I particularly delight in observing children instinctively dance to music. Toddlers, in particular, who can hardly stand yet, gleefully clap their hands and shake their booties at a wedding, a concert, or even during a musical TV commercial; evidence to me that we are all born with the music in us.

Write Your Story

I have no doubt, you already spice up your life with music. Since the selection of songs and arrangements is virtually infinite and your time is not, you're compelled to make choices. You can choose, for example, music that will move you to feel happy, energized, relaxed, sad or angry. Unlike any other time in history, you have all music from all time at your immediate disposal. You can wake up to the startling loud Buzzzzz of an alarm clock or be awaken to Norah Jones sweetly singing "Sunrise," obviously a smoother way to ease into the day. You can drive with a smile on your face and love in your heart singing praise songs or drive yourself into a state of road rage by blasting out angry rap tunes. You may select tunes that motivate, tunes that heal, or tunes that affect the way that you feel. The gift of music is yours for the choosing. Choose wisely, my friends.

Trust

What Science Says

Trust is vital to healthy relationships, whether it is the intimate relationship with our spouse or our more casual relationships with coworkers. Time, honesty, consistency, and being open about feelings are key factors in the development of trust. That trust can, however, be crushed in a moment. "It takes 20 years to build a reputation and five minutes to ruin it."[163] (Warren Buffett) Intuition may also be considered in deciding who to trust but, since intuition can be easily influenced by our past experience and current wants, it should be verified by tried and true friends over time and with the benefit of additional interactions. "Learning how to trust begins at birth: Babies are born completely dependent on caregivers to fulfill their basic needs for food, shelter, comfort, and love."[164] (Danielle Kassow at Thrive by Five Washington) "From an early age, children begin to differentiate between people who are trustworthy and those who aren't."[165] (researchers Melissa Koenig and Paul Harris) "Calm, consistent parenting creates an atmosphere of respect and trust in the family. Teens count on their parents to be there for them, even when setting up disciplinary consequences."[166] (child psychologist Russell Barkley) "Trust is about transparency, about learning that it's safe to let another person know who you are and what you feel, and it's basically trial and error. Trust is built when our partners have the opportunity to let us down or hurt us — but do not."[167] (Psychology Today) Coming from a family in which either or both parents were untrustworthy is a handicap to learning to trust or being trustworthy but it need not be a roadblock. It might just take a bit more communication, trial and error, understanding and compassion and a little more time. "The best way to find out if you can trust somebody is to trust them."[168] (Ernest Hemingway)

What God Says

God is trustworthy all of the time in every way. "He is absolutely sovereign over everything in the universe and He exercises that sovereignty in an infinitely wise and loving way for our good. If there is a single event in all of the universe that can occur outside of God's sovereign control, then we cannot trust him."[169] (Jerry Bridges in Trusting God) Although we, as God's children, may not always understand His wisdom, He reassures us, **"My plans are not like your plans, and my deeds are not like your deeds, for just as the sky is higher than the earth, so my deeds are superior to your deeds and my plans superior to your plans,"[170] (Isaiah 55:8-9)** and although God never promises that our lives will be pain free, **"we know that for those who love God all things work together for good."[171] (Romans 8:28)** God's children may enjoy the perfect peace that comes with deciding to **"Trust in the Lord with all our hearts, and do not lean on our own understanding. In all our ways acknowledge him, and he will make straight our paths. Be not wise in our own eyes; fear the Lord, and turn away from**

evil It will be healing to our flesh and refreshment to our bones."[172] (Proverbs 3:5-8)

One of My Stories

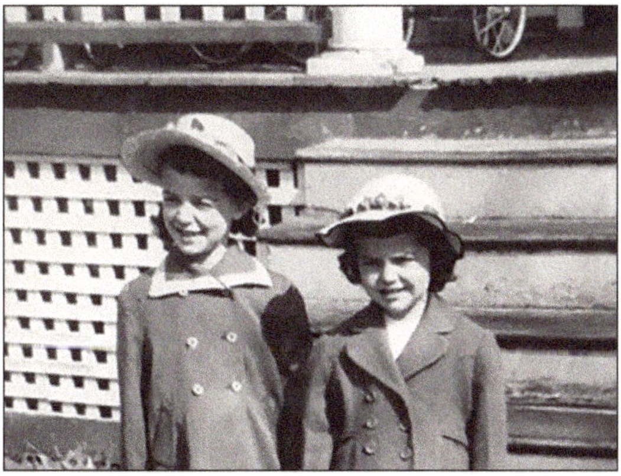

My sister Tisha and I are less than one and one half years apart in age. We shared a small bedroom, dolls, and spankings during our very young lives. We shared chores, clothes, and boys later on. We never had to worry about judgement or condemnation for anything we might divulge to each other. We are now privileged to enjoy the deep exhalation, shoulder dropping, face smiling kind of trust that develops over seven decades of consistently honest, compassionate, and respectful sharing of experiences and thoughts. Learning the fine art of trusting a spouse, for me, was quite another matter. Trust was not the hallmark of success for my first four failed marriages. The inability to trust was, at least contributory to their dissolutions. In

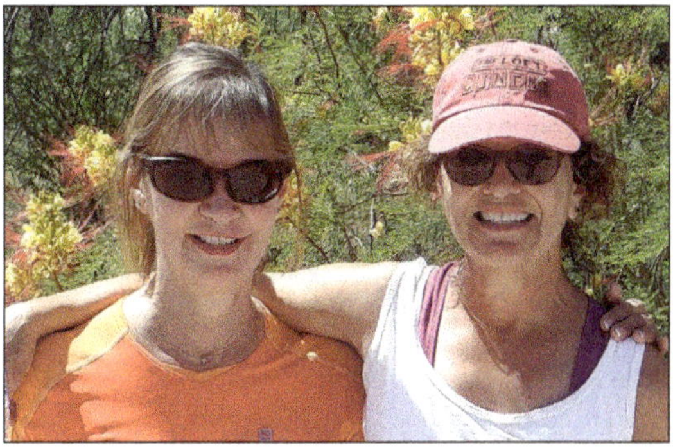

my current marriage, my husband and I put our trust first in God and then in each other. God's Word instructs us in how to love and trust openly and unselfishly. Since God is one hundred percent trustworthy and we are willing yet fallible, looking to God for direction keeps us on the same right path.

Write Your Story

First of all, beware not to err on the side of being too trusting. You may be tempted to trust too quickly that attractive person who is oh so charming or tells you just what you need to hear. This would be the time to step back and consult with your most reliable hard-nosed objective friend. How might you proceed then when someone, perhaps a member of your study group, asks you out for coffee? Since you have had a chance, through your group, to have observed their appearance, their treatment of others, their mannerisms and their opinions, trust yourself to make the decision about accepting the invitation. If, after meeting, no red flags are raised, and you find that you would like to get to know the person better, let the trust building begin. To build trust with your new friend, you need only to enjoy your time together in a consistently transparent, and respectful way. There is, however, no substitute for the tincture of time ingredient in the mix so make room for your ole pal "patience" to join the party. With God overseeing all my "parties," I count on His direction as to who to invite in and also who to invite back, knowing that only He is the sovereign event planner of this mega party called life.

Meditation

What Science Says

Ommmm. Most Americans aren't raised to sit cross legged with palms pointed up and chant "Om," but meditation has gained millions of converts, helping to ease chronic pain, anxiety, stress, improve heart health, boost mood and improve immunity. "Any condition that's caused or worsened by stress can be alleviated through meditation,"[173] says cardiologist Herbert Benson, MD, founder of the Mind/Body Institute at Harvard Medical School. Meditation is inhaling and exhaling it's way from the yoga studio into health clinics and schools with the primary effectiveness found in it's calming ability. Meditation is defined as "the act of giving attention to only one thing, either as a religious activity or just as a way of becoming calm and relaxed". Interestingly, spiritual meditation has been found to be superior to secular meditation in terms of decrease in anxiety and improvement in positive mood, spiritual health, spiritual experiences and tolerance to pain. As a religious activity, meditation is focused on listening for an answer from God. It is sometimes used synonymously with prayer. Although they do often go hand in hand, the two are distinctly different. Simply put, prayer is "speaking our desire" while meditation is "listening for the answer". Scientists have attempted to evaluate the effectiveness of prayer, finally reconciling that the rules for scientific study of the structure and behavior of everything are insufficient to measure the effectiveness of the Creator of everything. Galileo nicely described science's limits in the 1500's, "The aim of science is not to open a door to infinite wisdom but to set a limit to infinite error."[174]

What God Says

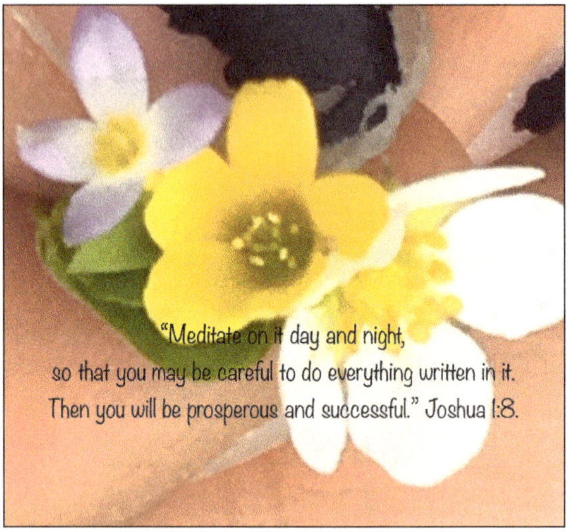

The Bible mentions "meditate" or "meditation" twenty three times, alone or combined with "prayer". God gave encouragement and instruction as the baton was passed from Moses to Joshua in leading God's people into the Promised Land, **"Keep this Book of the Law always on your lips; meditate on it day and night, so that you may be careful to do everything written in it. Then you will be prosperous and successful."[175] (Joshua 1:8)** The desired outcome of continued prayer and meditation is transformation. It is a means to a goal. Spending quiet time reading and meditating on God's Word leads to a **"peace that surpasses understanding."[176] (Philippians 4:7).**

One of My Stories

Five thirty a.m., off to the gym. Seven to eight, don't be late. Eight to four, patients galore. Four to nine, schoolwork and dine. Bed at ten, then do it again. I found no time to meditate, just a quick prayer then right out the gate. This was my life up to twenty years ago. In retrospect, God continued to beacon me at every juncture. It's been an evolution, on God's schedule, not mine. Getting to know Jesus better by studying the Bible became a desire of my heart. The "God of the Word" bible study was put in my path. I voraciously devoured Genesis through Exodus and have had an insatiable hunger for more ever since, recognizing the Bible as the only truth. I continue to be "transformed by the renewing of my mind." I still awaken at five thirty but, happily, the rest my routine has changed. I now give thanks for one more day, asking God to let me know what he wants me to do with what he has given me and to remove any interfering fears. Next, I cozy up on the couch with a hot cup of coffee and read a couple chapters of the Bible. This is followed by quiet prayer and meditation. To keep myself fit for duty, most days include exercise with a friend, then whatever work has been scheduled. I intentionally leave a time margin to fit it whatever additional or changed assignment God might lead me to. Throughout the day and before sleep, it's more talking with God (prayer) and listening (meditation). The prayer and meditation, for me, serve as a reset button, reminding me of what is important, that I am never alone, and that He will intercede when necessary. I have learned that I have a much better day when I hit the "reset" not just when I'm in trouble but as often as possible throughout the day. My practice of meditation has proven stress reducing and health promoting, although, in my case, causality cannot be attributed to meditation alone as it is always preceded by prayer.

Write Your Story

Contemplate your naval for twenty minutes and your blood pressure will decrease. Meditation, added to your daily routine, will reduce your stress and improve your health. Science has proven that. A more structured practice "mindful meditation," can be learned and it is touted to be even more effective. If you are ready to advance to the next therapeutic level, consider augmenting your meditation efforts with prayer. Even if you do not own a Bible, an easy starter method is to google on a topic you're interested in. If, for example, you are interested in health, google "bible and health." A list of various scriptural selections will appear. From the list, you might choose, for instance, the scripture, **"My child, pay attention to my words; listen attentively to my sayings. Do not let them depart from your sight, guard them within your heart; for they are life to those who find them and healing to one's entire body."**[177] **(Philippians 4:13).** Talk to God (prayer), and then, be still and listen(meditation).If other thoughts rudely interrupt, let them finish, then send them on their way and get back to the prayer at hand. Practice makes perfect. Meditation is good for your health. Add prayer and the possibilities are limitless.

Acceptance

What Science Says

"What we resist, persists."[178] (Carl Jung). Acceptance is necessary for our physical, emotional, and spiritual health. It is the acknowledgement that there is a situation or an emotion that is affecting us. It does not give the situation our seal of approval nor our consent for it to continue. What the research shows, and most of our experiences validate, is that "our willingness to accept the unchangeable has a great deal to do with our emotional and psychological well-being." Denial, the opposite of acceptance, is sometimes used as a survival stopgap when immediate acceptance would be just too painful, such as with the death of a loved one. "Denial is

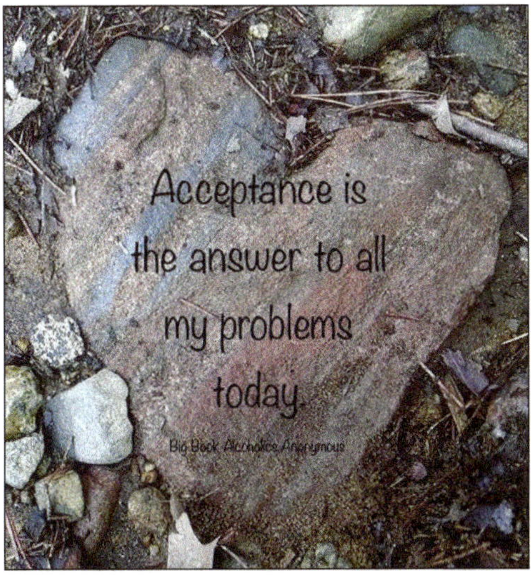

a coping mechanism that gives us time to adjust to distressing situations — but staying in denial can interfere with treatment or our ability to tackle challenges. Denial should only be a temporary measure — it won't change the reality of the situation."[179] (Mayo Clinic) Acceptance is key to healing. For the recovery of an alcoholic, for example, the Alcoholics Anonymous Big Book reads, "Acceptance is the answer to all my problems today. Until I could accept my alcoholism, I could not stay sober; unless I accept life completely on life's terms, I cannot be happy. I need to concentrate not so much on what needs to be changed in the world as on what needs to be changed in me and in my attitudes."[180] Achieving acceptance is a process; simple but not easy. Amy Morin, psychotherapist, author, and speaker, defines the process as, "acknowledging the problem, developing a plan, seeking help, changing what we can, identifying what we cannot change, and, finally, developing coping skills for taking care of ourselves."[181] Very often acceptance needs to be done in increments of moving forward and letting go. C.W. Lewis describes the process as "much like crossing monkey bars. You have to let go at some point in order to move forward."[182] (C.S. Lewis)

What God Says

When we, as Christians, accept that when problems are out of our control, God does have control and always wants the best for us, we experience the awesome gift of peace. The Bible tells us, **"Be still and know that I am God."[183] (Psalm 46:10)** the Bible makes known to us the importance of accepting and loving our neighbor by declaring it to be one of the two great commandments. **"Love the Lord your God with all your heart and with all your soul and with all your mind and "Love your neighbor as yourself."[184] (Matthew 22:36-40)** Jesus also makes it clear who our neighbor is, **"There is neither Jew nor Greek, there is neither slave nor free, there is no male and female, for you are all one in Christ Jesus."[185] (Galatians 3:28)** God abhors pride and the show of partiality. **"Everyone who is arrogant in heart is an abomination to the Lord; be assured, he will not go unpunished." (Proverbs 16:5) "For God shows no partiality."[186] (Romans2:11)** The last book of the Bible, Revelation, gives us a glimpse of those of us who will be forever residents of heaven and there is but one common denominator, acceptance of Jesus. **"After this I looked, and behold, a great multitude that no one could number, from every nation, from all tribes and peoples and languages, standing before the throne and before the Lamb, clothed in white robes, with palm branches in their hands, and crying out with a loud voice, "Salvation belongs to our God who sits on the throne, and to the Lamb!"[187] (Revelation 7:9-10)**

One of My Stories

The current civil unrest in America has brought my attention to the issue of "racism". In an attempt to define and accept this as a problem, I asked myself, "How can there be a problem between races when we are all members of one race, the human race?" This truism has always been declared by the Bible and is now proven and accepted as true by Science. Any differences seen between various communities of people are a result of genetics, geology and ethnicity. Historically, scientists, like Darwin, have mistakenly concluded that multiple levels of races exist, giving man's pride fuel to justify such atrocities as slavery, annihilation of the Jews, and exploitation of the American Indian, just to name a few. My heart grieves the pain this erroneous view of mankind has caused and still causes, not only to people of a particular skin pigmentation, but to all of us. Once again, pride is at the root of man's desire to feel "better than." God is abundantly clear about his abhorrence of pride and He repeatedly commands us to "love one another." This command to love includes people of all of the various melanin indices, different ethnicities, and different socioeconomic status. Now that I clearly see the current "racism" problem as yet another pride problem, I can accept it for what it is and "change the things I can." I confess that I have had experience with being prideful towards a particular group of people, namely those who seemed reluctant to work. After my guilt became sufficiently painful, I was convicted to ask God to help me with it. God must have really wanted me to change my heart because, within one day, a friend loaned me a book, "Bridges Out of Poverty" which led me to understand and feel compassion for the unemployed. God placed in my heart a desire to change the things I could change by contributing to the solution. I continue to ask God to show me areas where I may be prideful, to accept the problem, to solicit help, and to change the things I can change. Just so that I do not let a trouble causing prideful thought or action slide, I ask God to **"Search me, God, and know my heart; test me and know my anxious thoughts."[188] (Psalm 139:23)**

Write Your Story

It is often said that half the problem is knowing what the problem is. The next time you're feeling uncomfortably anxious but you do not know what is wrong, consider trying this. Take a time out and rerun your life from the time the discomfort started. Make note of what was occurring when the feeling of uneasiness occurred. Let's say, for example, that you recall that your son was very upset by the death of his pet fish one week ago. You were running behind schedule for work and school so you quickly addressed the situation by telling him you would buy him a new fish. After some thought and possibly consulting with your spouse, you realize and accept that the problem is perhaps your lack of supporting your son in grieving the loss of his pet fish. You cannot change that the fish has died and that you did not show empathy for your son's loss at the time. Forgive yourself then develop a plan to amend the situation. The plan might include spending time with your son to express your condolences for his loss, listening to him express his feelings and possibly offering to pick out a new fish together. Finally, enjoy following through on your plan. You would have successfully defined the problem, accepted the things you could not change, and changed the things you could. Your anxiety should then be replaced with serenity. If you have difficulty with any of the steps along the way, know that God loves to help out with these kinds of things when invited.

Pets

What Science Says

"Good dog." Dogs are very good indeed; good for our health and good for our happiness. Trisha McNair, MD, who has extensively studied the relationship between lifestyle and longevity estimates that dog ownership adds about two years to our life. "Having a dog is associated with a lower risk of death from cardiovascular disease or other causes," according to a study that followed 3.4 million people in Sweden. The study found that "for people who lived alone, owning a dog can decrease the risk of death by 33% and the risk of cardiovascular-related death by 36%, compared to single people without a pet. Chances of having a heart attack were also 11% lower."[189] "A 2019 review of nearly 70 years of research found that dog ownership lowers our risk of dying from any cause by 24%."[190] It's not just dogs that are beneficial, stroking our cats or any pet can lower our blood pressure and make us feel calmer. Even watching fish can relax us. Mayo Clinic finds that "animal-assisted therapy can

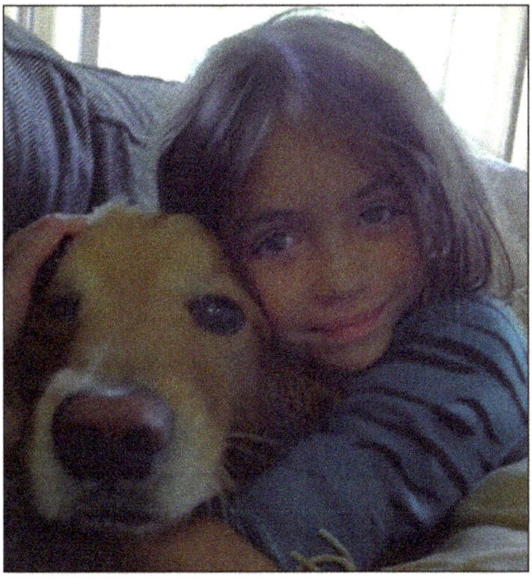

significantly reduce pain, anxiety, depression and fatigue in people with a range of health problems."[191] Physiologically it is the production of oxytocin, serotonin, and dopamine that promotes healing and health but anecdotally we can all attest to the "feel good" effect of hugging a big ole furry dog.

What God Says

To insure that the first created man, Adam, would have companionship, God created animals. He then made sure that Adam would bond with them by having him name each one. **"Then the Lord God said, "It is not good that the man should be alone; I will make him a helper fit for him." Now out of the ground the Lord God had formed every beast of the field and every bird of the heavens and brought them to the man to see what he would call them. And whatever the man called every living creature that was its name."[192] (Genesis 2:18-19)** After creating Eve as Adam's help mate, God then made Adam and Eve caretakers over the animals. **"Rule over the fish of the sea and the birds of the air and every creature that moves on the ground."[193] (Genesis 1:28)** God lovingly groups animals with humans as deserving of rest. **"Six days you shall do your work, but on the seventh day you shall rest; that your ox and your donkey may have rest, and the son of your servant woman, and the alien, may be refreshed.[194] (Exodus 20:9-11)** The Bible does not explicitly say that we will see our pets in heaven but it is written, **"And all flesh**

shall see the salvation of God,"[195] (Exodus 23:12) which I am hanging my leash on.

One of my Stories

I would never have been born if it were not for the love of a dog. My mother truly believed that my father married her to have someone at home to care for his navy dog's puppy, Chee Wee. I have been smitten for pups ever since, from Ripper to Blackie, to Maggie, to Chee Wee II, to Omar to Sleazy to Abbie to Moses and now to my ever so enthusiastic grand puppy, Porter. I can look forward, after an hour and a half drive, to being greeted by Porter's turning himself inside out to let me know that he has been counting the minutes until my arrival. He communicates through yelps and tail wags that no one pets him, talks to him, or throws a tennis ball like I do. He makes it known that if only I would

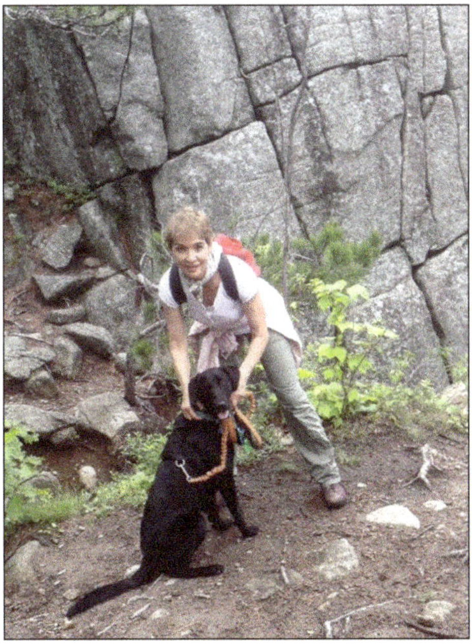

take him for a hike, his life would be complete. Even after I take over part of his spot on the couch or tire of throwing his tennis ball, no problem, he forgives me immediately. If I step out for coffee and return twenty minutes later, it's a celebration of long lost friends all over again. On the home front, my husband Fred does not let his cat allergy prevent him from enjoying a mutually beneficial relationship with two feral cats, Righty and Lefty. In exchange for their perceived input regarding their divergent political views, Fred prepares them custom meals from his stock of the best gourmet canned cat food mixed with select refrigerated left overs. Fred's health improves in his nurturing role and the kitties enjoy the finest of dining. It's a win win.

Write Your Story

Knowing that any amount of interaction with animals is mutually advantageous, you are limited only by your interest in a particular pet and your ability to care for it. If you must be away all day, cats are purr-rfic . They are independent with a litter box and bowls of water and food. You must, however, remember to earn their permission to live in their home. Dogs are all about pleasing you but do require more frequent feeding, toileting and attention. If you already have a pet, maximize your benefit by taking them on more walks, petting them more or practicing more sharing your thoughts and concerns with them. There's no need to own your own pet. You can enjoy your friend's and family's pets and, at the same time, share the care. We, and our pets, are designed to lovingly interact and mutually benefit. Pet, talk, walk.

Honesty

What Science Says

Honesty is the best policy. The truth will set you free. So then, why lie? People lie for a variety of reasons—to protect others, to protect themselves, or to benefit in some way. Honesty is not the normal state of affairs for most humans. Research from lying expert Robert Feldman suggests that "about sixty percent of us have a hard time getting through a ten-minute conversation without lying at least twice."[196] Another study estimates that the average person lies about eleven times a day. Lying, being selfish, cheating, and engaging in infidelity are associated with negative health outcomes such as elevated heart rate, increased blood pressure, vasoconstriction, elevated cortisol, and a significant depletion of the brain regions needed for appropriate emotional and physiological regulation. Not only does lying cause relationship difficulties, but in some situations, dishonesty may also

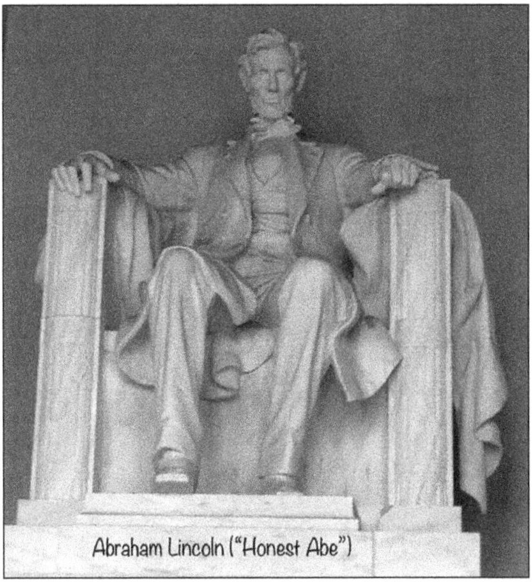

Abraham Lincoln ("Honest Abe")

lead to a tarnished reputation, career issues, and other social difficulties. When people lie, they then have to remember their lies in order to prevent them from being disproved. Aptly put by Honest Abraham Lincoln, "No man has a good enough memory to be a successful liar."[197] Often people have to tell additional lies to support the original lie resulting in an increasingly complicated series of lies that can be difficult to remember and stressful to manage. On the other hand, telling the truth is linked to an enhanced immune system, lower stress, decreased cellular aging, increased psychological well-being better friends, greater intimacy, and increased longevity of life.

What God Says

The Bible has a lot to say about the virtue of honesty with the denouncement of lying making number nine on the Ten Commandments; **"Thou shall not bear false witness. The Lord abhors a person who lies, but those who deal truthfully are his delight."[198] (Proverbs 12:22)** Being a God of truth and mercy, God commands that His followers not only show mercy by helping hurting people, but He, at the same time, requires they expose the things that hurt them so they can be led to the truth. The biblical metaphor, **"Where mercy and truth are met together; righteousness and peace have kissed each other."[199] (Psalm 85:10)** eloquently describes this command.

One of My Stories

A born liar, as are we all, I've worked at countering this noxious quality since it was revealed to me. Keeping this sinister snake from rearing its ugly head has taken continued diligence, sometimes, I have been told, to the point of offensiveness. In the last several years, God put people and circumstances in my life to help me grow in my approach to sharing my perceived truth with others. "Where is your mercy, lady?", my friend and colleague, Diane, asked after having witnessed me enlighten a client in the truth about their disease having been caused by their overeating. "You're enabling by being too soft with the truth," I retorted. "If they don't know the truth, they'll continue to over eat." After much thoughtful discussion and sharing of scripture and experiences, we each found ourselves converging toward a more middle ground approach, **"where mercy and truth are met together."(Psalm 85:10)** It is so important to me that I continue to present truth to others and to myself with a sufficient portion of mercy, that I have enlisted a few people close to me as accountability partners. My sister Tisha, as one, has agreed to be brutally honest with me if she observes me dishing out a helping of truth without a large enough scoop of mercy. It's a fine balance but, as everything good, it gets better with practice.

Write Your Story

When your good friend, Sweet Cakes, next asks the proverbial question, "Do I look fat in these jeans?" what will be your response? Do you blatantly lie so as not to hurt her feelings, while leaving her vulnerable to reprobate by others, or do you tell the raw truth? A third option might be for you to give your friend the benefit of a truthful response with a sufficient measure of mercy? You could say something like, "you are a beautiful person no matter what you wear but I remember seeing a style of jeans that would look even more fabulous on you." Then do the work to help her find them. Like many life practices, truth, wrapped in mercy when necessary, is more challenging in the short run but the long range benefit is the realization of freedom, improved health and more rewarding relationships.

Self Control

What Science Says

You are using self-control when you stop and think rather than react. If you think that reading this is in sync with your life goals, read on. "Self-control is the capacity to override one's impulse or desire in order to attain another goal."[200] (Mischel, 2014). It's what separates modern people from their ancient ancestors and the rest of the animal kingdom. Studies indicate that "self-control has wide-reaching implications for people's lives, including better physical health."[201] (Adler, 2015). One study by Seligman (2011) reported "self-control to be a major health asset with men with the highest self-control having a fifty six percent reduced risk for cardiovascular disease."[202] "Self-control better enables people to resist engaging in health-damaging behaviors, including the use of tobacco, alcohol, and other harmful substances."[203] (Miller et al. 2015) The alternative to exercising self-control is indulging in an action that momentarily satisfies a short-term goal at the expense of long-term rewards. Self-control can be improved with several key strategies. 1. Set clear life goals and keep them on the forefront of your mind as you go through your day, 2. Know that, like any other skill you want to master, self-control requires daily practice and repetition. 3. Go slow enough through your day that you recognize when you hit a frustrating moment. When you do hit a frustration challenge, stop. Push past the urge to react, instead, think. This is the opportunity for creativity and growth in self-control. Be aware that, like any change in behavior, it feels foreign and uncomfortable. With every subsequent success, your self-control, along with your self-esteem, will grow. You will become happier and healthier.

What God Says

In (Galatians 5:22-23) Apostle Paul lists nine attributes that are "the result of the work of the Holy Spirit in a Christian's life; love, joy, peace, forbearance, kindness, goodness, faithfulness, gentleness and self-control."[204] Self-control, specifically, is the ability to control one's body and its sensual appetites and desires – physically and mentally – through the power of the Holy Spirit. **The Bible instructs, "For the Spirit God gave us does not make us timid, but gives us power, love and self-discipline."[205] (2 Timothy 1:7)** It is empowering to know that we are not alone in this. It is the Holy Spirit within us that powers our own self-discipline to make, the right decisions regarding our health and welfare. Loving Father that he is, God always promises," **He will not let us be tempted beyond what we can bear. But when we are tempted, he will also provide a way out so that we can endure it."[206] (1 Corinthians 10:13)**

One of My Stories

Show me a lottery ticket and I'll walk right by. Drive a shiny new vehicle past me and I'll see a shiny new car payment. For me, the glitter and bling of movie stars and sports figures elicit yawns. I do, however, have my personal self-control nemesis. I walked into work a few days ago and there it was, all orange and yellow and sweet; a delectable bowl of the Halloween classic, candy corn. It was sweetly offered. It was plentiful and I was hungry. I stopped. I thought. Indulging in the candy corn was in conflict with several of my life goals, including good health. I felt transient discomfort and disappointment in walking by but oh so triumphant when I, alas, made it safely to my desk. In the past, I would have succumbed to an orgy of candy corn followed by an episode of sugar shock and near collapse. Instead, I got to enjoy another savory bite from the fruit of the spirit, self-control. The candy corn crisis, however, pales in comparison to experiences I've had of being on the receiving end of someone's decision to react with rage rather than choosing to control themselves by thinking first. The thought processes were the same, the impacts widely disparate. I remain confident that, with continued practice in the self control building process, anyone can improve and I believe that inviting God in on the process is the vital key to success.

Write Your Story

You've invested in a course at the local college as a step towards a degree in sociology. You've strategically completed your weekly and daily chores with plans to study for your first sociology exam. Just to make sure that there was no world situation you might be called on by the president to advise on, you decide to first watch the evening news. You learn that, yes, the earth is still spinning but then, "Breaking News". Coming up next is a, one time only, "Friends" Bingeathon. You, quick as lightening, sling that remote from your holster and aim point blank at the TV. You think, "Good grade and one step closer to a sociology degree or an evening of chuckles and nostalgia with Friends?" You shoot. A familiar discomfort is felt but you don't let it settle in. You may even make a quick call up for reinforcements, "God, need help here." After several hours of uninterrupted studying, you emerge from the books a conqueror. You look forward to your test with positive anticipation and with one step planted closer to your sociology degree goal. You flick on the TV and laugh to hear Joey still asking, "how YOU doin?" You doin just great.

Open Mindedness

What Science Says

Being open minded can be very good for our health, in that it allows in recommended strategies for improving our health which can then be rationally evaluated and put into practice. To be open minded means that we have a "willingness (or openness) to listen to, and perhaps even entertain, thoughts or ideas that may directly conflict with our already established beliefs."[207] (Cambridge Dictionary) Open mindedness is not the same as tolerance although they are often used interchangeably. Tolerance is defined as the "willingness to tolerate opinions or behaviors that one does not necessarily agree with."[208] It is fear that generally keeps the mind closed. "Often the fear is based on the idea that one must be right in order to be OK. It is not safe to be wrong. Therefore, once

"It is the mark of an educated mind to be able to entertain a thought without accepting it." (Aristotle)

an idea is grasped, one must hold on to it, for fear that to question it might prove one wrong and thus unsafe."[209] (Psychology Today) "People with a narrow perspective are more interested in proving themselves right than in getting the best outcome. They often focus much more on being understood than on understanding others."[210] ("Open Mindedness" by Wayne Riggs) We can broaden our world, open opportunity, and be a better problem solver by becoming more open minded. We can become more open minded by striving to become more approachable. Reading and sharpening our powers of observation increases opportunities to consider augmenting, modifying or affirming our current views and it gives us additional ideas to consider. An open minded interchange may be conducted by active listening, which always means less talking. The next step to becoming more open minded involves unfiltered thinking followed by research to verify information and to add additional data. Even if after a formal or informal analysis, we opt not to change or modify our current view, we will have had the opportunity to strengthen relationships or gain insights. "It is the mark of an educated mind to be able to entertain a thought without accepting it."[211] (Aristotle)

What God Says

God's Word, through the Bible, repeatedly teaches the merits of living with an open mind and firmly denounces close minded thinking. "**And the truth shall set you free."[212] (John 8:32.)** The "truth" is often interpreted to represent God who will set us free from worldly ignorance and the resultant unhealthy choices. **"A fool takes no pleasure in understanding but only in disclosing what is on his mind."[213] (Proverbs 18:2)** A "fool" is defined as "one who acts contrary to sound wisdom in his moral deportment; one who follows his own inclinations, who prefers trifling and temporary pleasure."[214] (Webster's Dictionary) God is not neutral on the suppression or the twisting of truth. **"For the wrath of God is revealed from heaven against all ungodliness and unrighteousness of men, who suppress the truth in unrighteousness, because what may be known of God is manifest in them, for God has shown it to them."[215] (Romans 1:18-19)** It has been my historical, as well as my personal, observation that if a person's mind remains open in pursuit of truth, that person is ultimately led to God.

One of My Stories

I had hit the proverbial "bottom" following a period of living in search of fitting in and being acceptable socially; the seductive possibilities of which were introduced to me through reentering the workforce. I remember thinking that "at last, I have discovered the way to achieve worldly sophistication and happiness." Finally, I could be a member of the "cool crowd." My mind was wide open but I was not discerning in what I chose to embrace; anything that the "in" people were doing, I considered worthy of emulating. I drank and cavorted my way to the loss of my marriage and loss of custody of my children. Years later, finding myself at an Alcoholics Anonymous meeting, I observed that the members who were happy, were those who professed faith in God. I tried to will some of this "faith" for myself but my "willing" was ineffective. I asked a few of these happy people how to will more effectively to get the prize, faith. They explained to me that, "willing" it does not work. You must pray for it by asking God to give it to you. I had had a past relationship with God and I could see that faith had clearly elevated a good number of members from the pit to peace so I decided to give prayer a try. I prayed for faith in God. My mind remained open waiting for results. At the same time, my brother John, seemingly out of the blue, reminded me that, as a child, I had accepted God's invitation for salvation and forgiveness of my sins. I strengthened my commitment by reaccepting. In very short order, faith hit me like a ton of bricks. I felt less alone and less afraid; also having been given, what I now recognize, as hope. Having experienced the transforming effects of prayer and faith, I developed a thirst for more which I quenched through studying God's Word, the Bible. I approached, and continue to approach my study with an open mind; inquisitive, challenging, and rational. In the case of my faith, the open minded approach has caused my faith to strengthen. Having a firm base of belief facilitates the welcoming, the processing, and the responding to new information and ideas in a non-threatening, analytical manner. With my roots now firmly planted in healthy soil, I am well positioned to thrive and to grow.

Write Your Story

A truly open mind is a very good thing. It makes your life larger and more exhilarating and provides a path for personal growth. I caution you, however, to beware of deception. A healthy open mind does not assimilate just any idea that come along into your life, does not automatically go along with the crowd, and does not confuse open mindedness with tolerance. You can enjoy being open minded, in a healthy way, by listening well, studying the facts, thinking, and respectfully discussing an issue. What you have to gain, at most, is new information, insights, or the refining of current beliefs. At very least, you gain greater understanding and respect for those you interact with in the process. Try it. Say that, if today, your child comes home on his first break from college and announces, "I have decided not to pursue medicine. I have met my soul mate, Linda Lace, and we are quitting school to save the whales." You may consider offering up a quick prayer for this one. Lovingly listen, listen, listen. Perhaps offer to research the several options together; a quick marriage now vs a nice wedding later, or perhaps using a potential physician's salary down the road to save even more whales. Maybe take time out for individual thinking, then get back together to respectfully discuss the options again in a unconditionally loving way. There is never a guaranteed outcome but, at the very least, an open mind will keep communication open and save the relationship.

Journaling

What Science Says

When C.S. Lewis lost his beloved wife, journaling was the only thing he found strong enough to kill the pain. "But what am I to do? I must have some drug, and reading isn't a strong enough drug now."[216](C.S. Lewis). Although journaling has always been recognized as a potent mediator of emotional pain, science has now proven it. What science found was that "when we put our feelings into words, we reduce the response in the amygdala while activating the brains prefrontal region, making the feelings less intense."[217] (UCLA psychologists) Journaling, though it takes a few minutes to do, is actually a time saver and an effective tool for healthy living. Putting our thoughts on a simple piece of paper, or a paper equivalent, actually "frees up our brain matter to do other things,"[218] according to research from Baylor University's Sleep Neuroscience and Cognition Lab. Writing can make us better people. "Expressive writing noting feelings of gratitude has demonstrated to lead to an upward swing in selfless generosity."[219] (University of Oregon research). Journaling is the "write" remedy for insomnia. Thanks to research from Baylor University's Sleep Neuroscience and Cognition lab, evidence that writing a to-do list to 'offload' thoughts and reduce worry is no longer merely anecdotal. Using overnight polysomnography, researchers found that "subjects who wrote out a to-do list prior to sleep fell asleep faster than those who journaled about completed tasks."[220] Journaling is proven to enhance overall health. University of Texas at Austin psychologist and researcher James Pennebaker contends that "regular journaling strengthens immune cells, called T-lymphocytes." Other research indicates that "journaling decreases the symptoms of asthma and rheumatoid arthritis." The merit of journaling in creative problem solving is also backed by research. "The act of writing accesses your left brain, which is analytical and rational. While your left brain is occupied, your right brain is free to create, intuit and feel. Writing removes mental blocks and allows you to use all of your brainpower to better understand yourself, others and the world around you. Typically we problem solve from a left-brained, analytical perspective. But sometimes the answer can only be found by engaging right-brained creativity."[221] (James Pennebaker) How to journal is as varied as it's benefits; the only requirement is that you do it. It can be regular or it can be sporadic. It can be mixed content or subject based. However your journaling is born and evolves, it can be a faithful and true teacher and friend. You may want to consider your grammar and legibility for future reference. Publication of one particular young journalist's thoughts, was translated to seventy different languages and sold over thirty million copies. She humbly wrote, "It seems to me that later on neither I nor anyone else will be interested in the musings of a thirteen-year old school girl. Oh well, it doesn't matter. I feel like writing."[222] (Anne Frank)

What God Says

There is a particular compilation of journals that has withstood the test of time and has had massive influence on the world. It is referred to as "The Bible." The entire Bible is God inspired, pen put to paper by forty men of varied educations and backgrounds over a span of fifteen hundred years. **Thus says the Lord, the God of Israel: Write in a book all the words that I have spoken to you."[223] (Jeremiah 30:2)** It contains pure and timeless truth about God, about life, and about the nature of mankind. It is the only book of antiquity which has proven to be true by history, by modern sciences, and by the fulfillment of its prophesy. The Bible is a historical journal beginning with the story of the creation of man. It is a how to live life instruction manual, and it is the only book that has withstood the test of time for validity. King David demonstrated wisdom in studying and meditating on the Bible. **"I will meditate on your precepts and fix my eyes on your ways."[224] (Psalm 119:15)** We would be wise to do the same. Journaling is a traditional and an effective tool for doing so.

One of My Stories

One of my childhood treasures was a mint green diary with a small gold key. The pages were thick and shiny and it had a "new book" smell. I do not recall anything that I wrote in it but I do remember the pleasure of unlocking it and locking it back up. Since then, I have benefited from various forms of journaling. In writing out classroom notes, sometimes several times, I learned to be effective in bumping up my test scores, later delighting in learning that this phenomena was supported by research. “Feelings” journals, when reviewed at a later date, made it abundantly clear to me how flagrantly erratic my feelings were depending on the time of the month or how much sugar I had consumed. The circumstances and the other parties involved were secondary, teaching me a valuable lesson about myself and about human nature in general. I was amazed and comforted by reviewing my bible study group’s weekly prayer journal at the end of the semester. I learned how many and in which ways the prayers of group members had been answered. I have learned to use my very smart phone to “journal” to-do’s that invariable come to mind at days end. This allows me to release the day and drift off. Through trial and error, I have settled into using a purse size journal to record ideas, insights, scripture, must reads, or experiences that may be useful for inspiration, meditation, education or just because. I now realize that I fortuitously chose mint green.

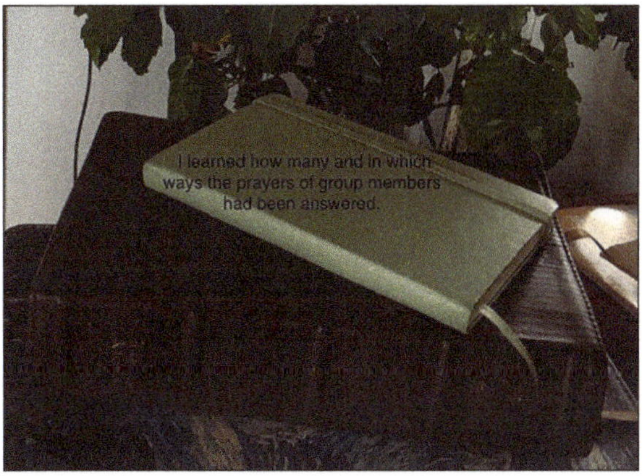

Write Your Story

Knowing that time invested in journaling yields a high return, why not grab a pen and a notebook then say hello to your new nonjudgmental, open armed friend. Giving yourself privacy, write freely and without self-censor. There will be no grading so do not worry about spelling, grammar, or punctuation. The only rule is, there are no rules. Now let your mind flow onto the paper. If you are stressed, let the paper have it. If you're conflicted or confused, write it down. Read it back now and read it back later. You can be your own highly paid consultant, looking at problems anew and creatively solving them. If you are having a disagreement, writing it down can give you the objectivity needed to come up with a resolution. Gift yourself praise for accomplishments, expressions of gratitude and hopes for the future. At intervals, reminisce with your journal friend by looking back at past entries, commending yourself for growth and reliving fond memories, keeping in mind that this friend is you. "Fill your paper with the breathings of your heart."[225] (William Wordsworth)

Faith

What Science Says

Medical science supports the commonly accepted view that people of faith are both happier and healthier. Measurable indicators include a longer lifespan, and a lower rate of depression and suicide. In addition, a review of 250 epidemiological health research studies found a reduced risk of colitis, different types of cancer, and untimely death among people with higher levels of faith. Another important indicator, an increased resilience found with people of faith, is vital to everyone's health but is absolutely essential to the spiritual, emotional and physical health of children and teens. Faith gives people a sense of meaning and purpose in life, which is linked to better health, while secularism sucks the peace out of people because they have no way of coping with life's fears. Faith is defined as a complete trust or confidence in someone or something. If that someone or something is steadfast and solid, the health benefits are not only significant, but are commensurate with the degree of faith.

What God Says

God is the most steadfast and solid being in this whole universe. **"Trust in the Lord with all your heart, and do not lean on your own understanding. In all your ways acknowledge him, and he will make straight your paths."[226] (Proverbs 3:5-6)** God repeatedly tells us, thru his Word, that, **"He is our refuge, our one place of security, our hope in the face of the uncertainties. He is our Rock!"[227] (Psalms 18:2).** In other words, if we have complete trust that an all-powerful God has our best interests at heart and will always show us the best way to go if we but ask, we have effectively passed the weight of the world from our shoulders to His.

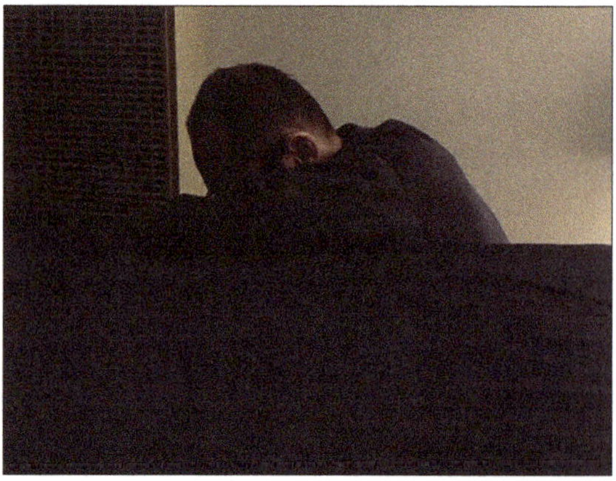

One of my Stories

Ignoring the "me first" worldly financial advise and deciding, in faith, to obey the tithing instruction I had recently learned from the Bible, within three years my financial situation changed from red to black. My financial savvy inexplicably upgraded and my fear about having enough money dissipated. I was no longer in it alone. The weight on my shoulders lifted just a bit and the next little leap of faith was easier. Every time I hand a situation over to God in faith, the freer and likely the healthier I become.

Write Your Story

Health results from building a life on solid ground. If you're experiencing disease or at least unease by placing your faith in a fickle, seductive, and precarious world, consider upgrading your foundation. He's right there, a solid rock of love and truth, gently knocking with an offer to lighten your load and be right there with you and for you. It only takes faith the size of a mustard seed to take that first step. You've nothing to lose; improved health and forever happiness to gain.

Sleep

What Science Says

Americans currently average 6.8 hours of sleep at night, down more than one hour from 1942 and far below the seven to nine hours recommended. With one in five adults failing to get enough sleep, the impact on morbidity and productivity is significant. Sleep helps us thrive by contributing to a healthy immune system, and can also balance our appetites by helping to regulate levels of the hormone leptin. Medical studies have related a lack of sleep to physical health problems such as heart disease and diabetes and mental disorders such as depression, anxiety, and substance abuse. Any true insomniac worthy of dark circles and droopy eyelids knows the primary cause of his wakefulness, the big W, Worry. We lay awake or awaken to mull over things that can only be made more challenging by facing them exhausted. Science gives recommendations for insuring a good night's sleep. We're advised to keep bedtime and wake time consistent, to exercise early in the day, to limit caffeine and alcohol, to avoid nicotine and to avoid large evening meals. It is also advised that we create a dark, cool and comfortable bedroom, that we develop a regular bedtime ritual and that our bedroom is used only for sex and sleep. If the the worry and "to do" list is transferred to a hard copy and the available space in your head is replaced with a gratitude list, the chance of drifting off is significantly increased.

What God Says

Jesus recommends another option for worry and insomnia. He tells us how to rest. **"Come to me, all of you who are weary and carry heavy burdens, and I will give you rest. Take my yoke upon you. Let me teach you, because I am humble and gentle at heart, and you will find rest for your souls."[228] (Matthew 11:28-29)** When we accept Jesus into our hearts, we can have the peace of knowing that **"When we lie down, we will not be afraid; when we lie down, our sleep will be sweet."[229] (Psalm 127:2)** He invites us to hand over our worries to him. This is so important to Him that we know this that it's mentioned over 365 times in the Bible. God modeled the practice of rest for us on day seven of creation. After creating the universe and it's earthly inhabitants, including man and woman, God stood back, admired his work and rested. We can be quite confident, that God, who spoke the world into existence, did not rest because he was pooped out from the arduous task of creating you or I or for lack of proper conditioning. He was modeling a lifestyle for us; periods of work followed by rest.

One of My Stories

If there's anything I'm an expert at, it's the fine art of worrying. Around two a.m., I would combine my imagination, projection, and recollection skills to provide an infinite supply of worry material sufficient to keep me awake for weeks. Most nights now I sleep in peace.

A quiet, dark, cool room and a comfy bedroom is basic. I enjoy a healthy diet, exercise, avoidance of toxins, and do aim for a regular sleep schedule, awaking naturally every day at 5:30. Just before retiring, to change my focus from my worldly perspective, I meditate on a little scripture from the Bible. I then hand over to God the worries I may have taken back during the day and, instead of counting sheep, I count blessings as I melt into sleep. In addition, since I have deliberately taken Sundays as a day of rest, my energy level and my productivity for the week has increased.

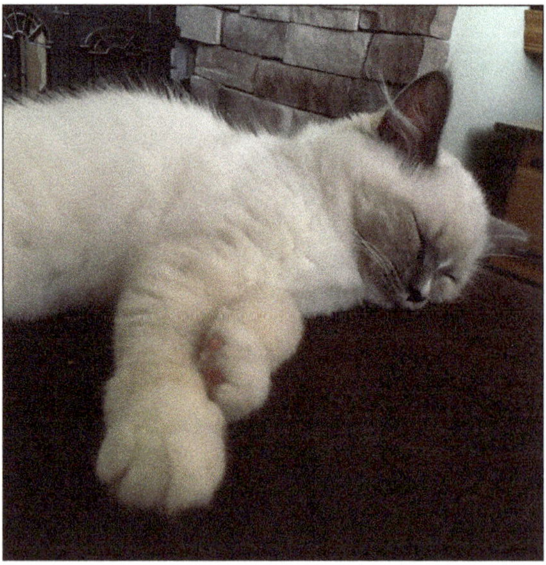

Write Your Story

Are you resisting a rest? A peaceful night's rest can be yours but don't expect it to happen overnight. Consider starting your improved sleep hygiene by establishing a wake up time and sticking to it. Have fun creating a sleep inviting bedroom and a pleasant sleep routine. Try a spot of Sleepytime tea and a warm lavender bath perhaps, or whatever suits your personal fancy. It would be a powerful next step to hand over your worries. (You can always grab them back in the morning) then settle in to count your blessings. Awe come on, you do have blessings. Just get started. If you cannot sleep within 20 minutes or so, no problem. Get up and read in the next room until you're sleepy then back to bed and start counting. Sweet dreams.

PERSISTENCE

What Science Says

IF YOUR GOAL IS TO BE SUCCESSFUL, "Nothing in the world can take the place of persistence. Talent will not; nothing is more common than unsuccessful men with talent. Genius will not; unrewarded genius is almost a proverb. Education will not; the world is full of educated derelicts. Persistence and determination alone are omnipotent."[230] (Calvin Coolidge) This opinion is shared by a multitude of renown thinkers. Albert Einstein offers a humble, simplistic, summation, "It is not that I'm so smart. But I stay with the questions much longer."[231] Martin Luther King Jr. speaks to the tenacity of persistence, "If you can't fly then run, if you can't run then walk, if you can't walk then crawl, but whatever you do you have to keep moving forward."[232] We need not give up on achieving success if we seem to be lacking in persistence. "The ability to create a habit of persistence or perseverance isn't something reserved for a few—it is available to you!" According to behavioral scientist Dr. Jean Wiechai, "perseverance involves consciously developing a routine, sticking to it, and consciously rewarding yourself for each completed goal, however small."[233] Studies show that each time we reward ourselves for acting towards accomplishing a goal, our endocrine system doses out a dopamine reward, thus reinforcing the action. After several repetitions, a habit of perseverance is strengthened. Persistence building has proven effective where other approaches have failed in programs such as Alcoholics Anonymous's "One Day at a Time" method of alcohol abstinence and Nike's "Just do it!" approach to exercise. You too can do it too but "if you don't succeed the first time, try and try again."

What God Says

God, the Perfect Father, instructs his children in becoming successful followers of Christ through persistence "**And let us not grow weary of doing good, for in due season we will reap, if we do not give up."[234] (Romans 5:3-5)** He further advises us that even our suffering can be seen as a good thing if it develops our persistence, **"we rejoice in our sufferings, knowing that suffering produces endurance, and endurance produces character, and character produces hope."[235] (Philippians 3:14)** Jesus modeled extreme persistence in enduring persecution while focusing on his goal of paying for our ticket to heaven.

One of My Stories

Reading Calvin Coolidge's proclamation on the value of persistence was a eureka moment for me, helping to make some sense of the course of my life. Growing up in a resource challenged environment gave me a considerable advantage in developing persistence. Because I wanted to wear cool clothes to school, I was motivated to persevere in sewing my own clothes. To realize a desire to live in a designer bedroom, I learned to refurbish furniture, paint, and paper while developing a knack for design. Projects were financed by perfecting the Dairy Queen ice cream signature swirl top and later by scooping all 28 flavors of Howard Johnson's ice cream. This financial need to work born in me a useful work ethic, of which persistence is a requisite component. At some point, I answered God's invitation to share my challenges with him. Since then, my persistence has become super charged, with knowing well in my heart that **"with God all things are possible."** My son has followed a similar path and with the same spiritual connection. He persevered through college while playing football then rescued and grew a failing business he took on through a recession. Tackling each major challenge and sub challenge head on developed in him a habit of persistence that did not stop when circumstances improved. He was ultimately inspired

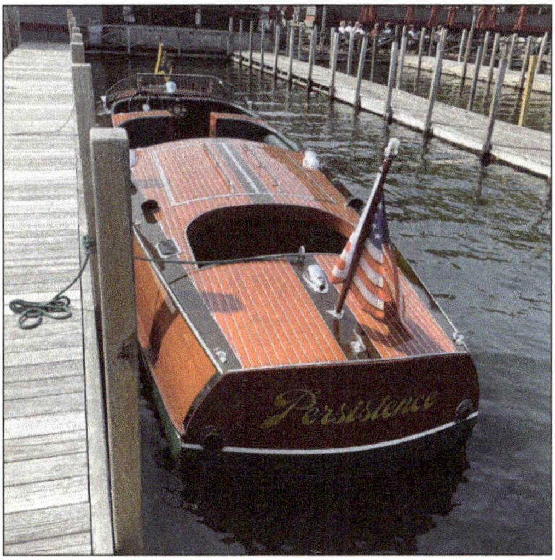

to name one of his boats "Persistence," which is docked in front of one of his homes. Most importantly, he and I have learned that when persistence is God powered, anything is possible.

Write Your Story

Since persistence is key to success at reaching any goal, why not use it towards a goal of improved health and happiness? If your plan is to start exercising, for example, you might start by telling a few people your plan. You may then decide to set out your spiffy exercise clothes the night before. In the morning, you ignore the urge to smother the alarm and roll over in bed and, instead, you arise. Ta Da! You've just accomplished the most difficult step. Reward yourself with a heartfelt compliment which will trigger a reinforcing hit of dopamine. As you exercise, you smile and tell yourself, "This is fun! I like it and I am doing it! You repeatedly reward yourself with positive self-talk throughout the day; more dopamine, more habit reinforcement. "Just do it" "one day at a time" for six more weeks and your persistence will not only be rewarded with positive self-talk but you will be further rewarded by improved health and happiness. Feel perfectly entitled to use your enhanced skill of persistence to conquer the world. If you find your personal power to be at all insufficient, you might do as I do, invite in God's power.

Smile

What Science Says

"Smile and the world smiles with you; frown and you frown alone." This is not only a catchy song lyric but it's credibility is backed by research. If you're smiling at someone, they can't help but smile back. In fact, not smiling back takes conscious effort. "The part of your brain that is responsible for your facial expression of smiling when happy or mimicking another's smile resides in the cingulate cortex, an unconscious automatic response area of the brain. When you smile at someone, you are creating a symbiotic relationship that allows both of you to release feel-good chemicals in your brain, activate reward centers, make you both more attractive, and increase the chances of you both living longer, healthier lives. Smiling is also proven to activate the release of neuropeptides that work toward fighting off stress. The feel-good neurotransmitters—dopamine, endorphins and serotonin—are all released when a smile flashes across your face as well. This not only relaxes your body, but it can also lower your heart rate and blood pressure. The serotonin release brought on by your smile also serves as an anti-depressant/mood lifter."[236] (Ronald E Riggio Ph.D. Cutting-Edge Leadership) There's no need to feel joy to initiate a smile. "Sometimes your joy is the source of your smile, but sometimes your smile can be the source of your joy." [237] (Thich Nhat Hanh)

What God Says

God's children, who are filled with the fruits of the spirit, are more likely to present with a joyful continence, often expressed with a smile. I envision Jesus, while walking among us, smiling as he went about healing and ministering. **"The Son of Man came, enjoying life"[238] (Matthew 11:19)** The Bible tells us numerous times that a smile is good for our health. **"A happy heart makes the face cheerful, but heartache crushes the spirit."[239] (Proverbs 17:22)** Smiling is one of the qualities of an "excellent wife" described in the book of Proverbs, **"Strength and dignity are her clothing, And she smiles at the future."[240] (Proverbs 31:25)** God's commands can be summarized in two sentences, **"Love God. Love Each Other."** A smile is reflection of both.

One of My Stories

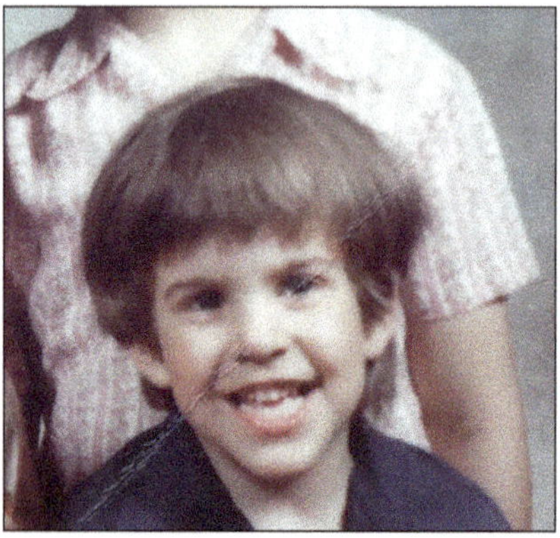

"He smiled from the day he was born," I always said of my son, Chris. Every child is born with a unique temperament. Chris's temperament was easy going with a ready smile. As a toddler, he was easily brought to laugher by his older brother Rob and, together, they found it hysterically amusing to tease their younger sister Angela. As a teen, Chris's family, myself included, were so accustomed to his antics, that we would smile and prepare to laugh as soon as he walked in the door. Chris would

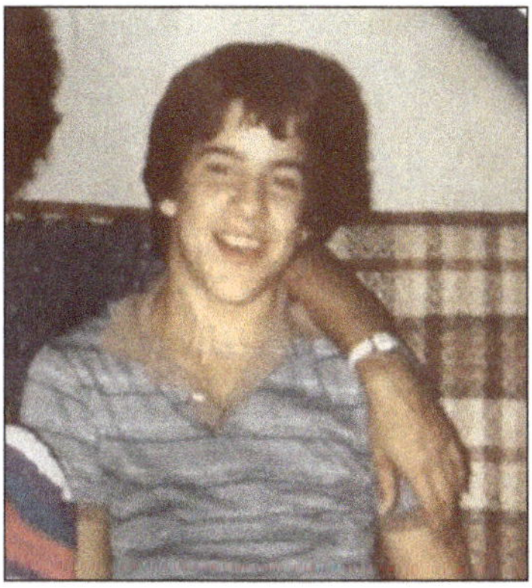

go to any length to make people laugh, whether precariously surfing on the icebergs as the Lake George ice broke up or doing hand stands on his classroom desk. His smile and personality were magnets, attracting family and friends alike. I knew Chris to have the tender heart of an old soul. I hold tight to the memory of Chris's bus driver telling me how, Chris intentionally sat with the little girl on the elementary school bus who no one else would sit with.

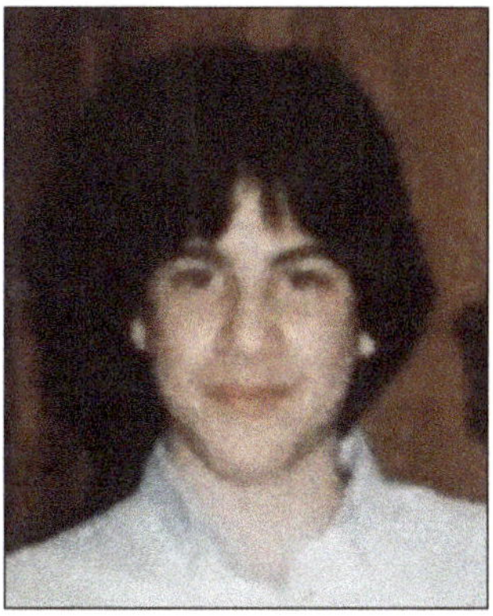

Years later, as a burly football jock, Chris left his band of cronies to sit with me at a sports ceremony after he noticed I had arrived alone. All he did, he did with a smile on his face, reflecting the warmth in his heart. When he passed to his eternal residence on August 17, 1990, those close to him all agreed with the message to be placed on Chris's Memorial Stone, "Chris's ministry is his smile, his enthusiasm, and his friendship." To honor Chris, I strive to share his ministry.

Write Your Story

Why not, this week, launch your own personal smile challenge? Knowing that whenever you smile at a person, their brain actually coaxes them to return the favor, you can be confident of a returned smile. Whether or not, your targeted smilee smiles back, your body will produce feel good, and health enhancing chemicals and you will look even more marvelous, darling. Most likely, your smile receiver will smile back and you will both win. Keep smiling. Those around you will see you as friendly, intelligent, and attractive. As a bonus, "Smiling makes people wonder what you're up to."[241] Jill Shalvis

Hope

What Science Says

We can survive 40 days without food, three days without water, and eight minutes without air but we cannot last a single second without hope. It is an essential part of life. When hope is gone, life is over. It has been challenging to come up with a universally accepted definition of hope upon which to base this discussion. Webster defines hope as a "feeling of expectation and a desire for certain thing to happen."[242] Psychologist Charles Snyder and colleagues expand the definition to include the "will to get to a goal and having different ways to get there."[243] Neuroscientists have demonstrated that a feeling of hopefulness changes your brain. Hope, which involves belief and expectation, causes the brain to release chemicals called endorphins and enkephalins which actually mimic the effects of morphine. The result is that the brain can overcome hurdles and moves to a place of recovery. Science explains the "source of hope as rooted in unalloyed reality. Hope is the elevating feeling we experience when we see – in the mind's eye – a path to a better future." According to Jerry Groopman, MD, in his book, The Anatomy of Hope. "Hopelessness is a strong predictor of adverse health outcomes, independent of depression and traditional risk factors, and increases mortality and the incidence of myocardial infarction and cancer,"[244] whereas, hope is credited as the common denominator among survivors, achievers and reformers.

What God Says

In the Bible, hope is the confident expectation of what God has promised and its strength is in His faithfulness. "Hope isn't the same as optimism. It isn't the belief that something bad will turn out well. It is the absolute confidence that every part of your life ultimately makes sense, regardless of how it turns out this side of eternity,"[245] according to Pastor Rick Warren. People everywhere are looking for hope in all the wrong places. They look for it in their relationships, in self-help books, and in self-righteousness, but there is only one place to find real hope. The Bible says real hope is found by turning to God: ***"May God, the source of hope, fill you with joy and peace through your faith in him. Then you will overflow with hope by the power of the Holy Spirit"[246] (Romans 15:13)*** Hope, sometimes confused with faith, is different than faith in that faith says it is so now, and hope says in the future it could happen.

One of My Stories

For the first six decades of my life, my hope level waxed and waned with my degree of confidence in whatever relationship, contemporary expert, or self-direction I was leaning on. Being a product of an unpredictable alcoholic family system, and having found reward in the academic realm, for me, the most reliable source for providing the how to for achieving my goals was education. Hope soared with worldly achievement and plummeted with even the smallest of disappointment. I would briefly float on cloud nine when selected for a job position, for example, but would drop to the pits if I was not immediately promoted to CEO. I was up after becoming engaged to Prince Charming but quickly in the doldrums when he raised his voice to me. I had not lost the desire part of the hope equation but the confidence in my ability to get there was unstable at best, having built it on a foundation of my own making. It wasn't until I came to believe that a power greater than myself, God, could provide an unshakable foundation, did I learn what real hope felt like. I now had, not only the desire, but also the steadfast promises of a God who ***"works all thing for the good."*** to rely on. The belief that ***"With God all things are possible."*** is factored into every decision I make. I am in no way saying that I live a life of unending lollipops and roses. I face many pitfalls and experience much sadness along the way, but I do maintain a hope founded on solid bedrock, looking forward to whatever is in my future knowing that He will provide whatever I need. I believe his promise,

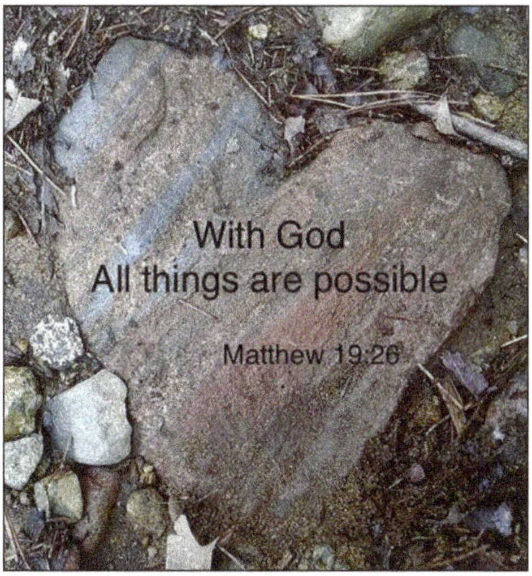

"My heavenly Father already knows all my needs. Seek the Kingdom of God above all else, and live righteously, and he will give me everything I need"[247](Matthew 6:32-33)

Write Your Story

How hopeful are you about your life and your future? Imagining the fulfillment of your dreams and goals and having plans with several contingencies for reaching your goals will boost your hope level and contribute to a healthier happier you. Building goal achieving confidence by reminding yourself of past successes also enhances your sense of hope. If you would really like to super charge your hope, you could step up and start building it on the Rock. I hope you do.

Patience

What Science Says

"One moment of patience may ward off great disaster. One moment of impatience may ruin a whole life."[248] (Chinese Proverb). Impatience, defined as "feeling and showing hostility towards, or about, things which obstruct, frustrate or delay one's goals,"[249] is most often negative but it is not always a bad thing. Patience is defined as "the capacity to accept or tolerate delay, trouble, or suffering without getting angry or upset."[250] As with many attributes, it is at least somewhat about the balance and the control as to how useful or detrimental it might be. "If we are too patient, we can waste vast stretches of our lives pursuing the wrong goals."[251] (Psychology today). We might decide, for instance, that after many months of training and many bruises and muscle strains, our time might be better spent, at age seventy, at something other than becoming a professional gymnast. On the other end of the spectrum, too much impatience can significantly affect our health. In their 2007 study, Schnitker and Emmons found that "patient people were less likely to report health problems like headaches, acne flair-ups, ulcers, diarrhea, and pneumonia."[252] Other research has found that "people who exhibit impatience and irritability tend to have more health complaints and worse sleep." How does the impatience reaction happen? Simply put, impatience is triggered when the cost of achieving our goal exceeds our expectations. If we find that impatience is causing harm in our lives, know that our patience muscle can be developed, the process very similar to the development of our physical muscles. Jim Stone, PhD makes some practical recommendations. "Take a deep breath. Identify which goal is being frustrated. Identify how the perceived costs of reaching that goal have risen. Decide, calmly and rationally, whether you should 1) try to find a shortcut, 2) switch goals, or 3) settle in and come to peace with the situation. If you have decided to settle in and come to peace with the situation, then accept the increased costs, and change your mindset."[253] Say, for example, I am spreading mulch in my garden, which I expect to complete before the rain starts in two hours. My neighbor stops by with the gift of warm home baked cookies and wants to discuss the neighborhood association. The time cost of reaching my goal now exceeds my expectation and I sense an itchy trigger finger on the impatience button. While politely sampling a cookie, I take a deep breath and work the decision for patience process through in my head. I ultimately change my mindset to one of enjoying a conversation with my gourmet neighbor and looking forward to the fun of mulching in the rain. As with any muscle development, it gets stronger and easier with practice and, in time, "muscle memory", will make patience an automatic reaction to a challenge to our goals.

What God Says

Patience holds a high place in the lives of God's children. It is actually listed as one of the **fruits of the spirit along with love, joy, peace, kindness, goodness, faithfulness, gentleness, and self-control."[254] (Galatians 5:22)**, all valuable assets individually and even better when in combination. We are instructed to do everything God leads us to do with great patience, **"Preach the word; be prepared in season and out of season; correct, rebuke and encourage—with great patience and careful instruction."[255] (2 Timothy 4:2)** "The human instinct is to cry out to God in bewilderment when tribulation comes knocking. We blame. We resist. We complain. What we don't do is say, Thank You, Father; it is time to grow in patience. People are not trained to think that way but, according to the Bible, that is exactly how Christians are to respond. Accepting hardship as a means of growth is a radical concept in this world. Even more extreme is the believer who praises the Lord for the storm. But God's followers have cause to rejoice. Tribulation increases our patience so that we can stand firm on His promises and await His good timing."[256] (Charles Stanley) God, through scripture, raises the bar by telling us to be patient even with difficult people. **"The Lord's servants must not quarrel but must be kind to everyone. They must be patient with difficult people."[257] (2 Timothy 2:24)** Impatience is described as a most undesirable quality, **"Do not let yourself be quickly provoked, for anger resides in the lap of fools."[258] (Ecclesiastes 7:9)** For the welfare of each individual child of God and for mankind as a whole, developing and practicing patience is essential.

One of My Stories

The cat is touted to be the symbol of patience, known for its ability to wait and act only when the time is right. I will demonstrate this positive feline quality in the story of Miss Kitty and Moses. Miss Kitty, a beautiful tortoise shell kitty was left in my care when her adoptive mama, my daughter Angela, went off to college.

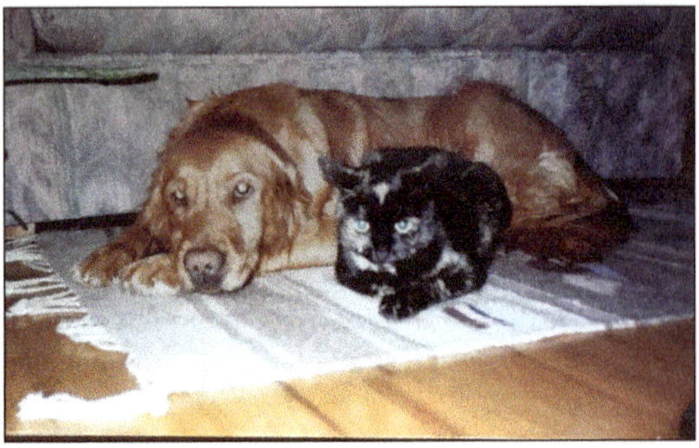

As a college cat, Miss Kitty felt herself well qualified to dictate the behavior of her, then, older sister Abigail, the Golden Retriever. In exchange for sliding the screen door open so that Abigail could escape, Abigail allowed Miss Kitty to use her luxuriously soft body for her personal mattress. At Abigail's passing at age fifteen, Miss K took it very hard, as did we all. When Moses, the German Shepherd, was adopted into the household, Miss K assumed that he would also accommodate her need for a soft warm canine bed. Much to Miss K's chagrin, Moses ascribed to the traditional "dogs rule cats," dogma. Over time, Moses became accustomed to sleeping on the lower corner of my bed. After several weeks of rejection by Moses, Miss K unobtrusively poised herself on the other corner of the bed. Over the course of seven years, Miss K gradually inched herself closer and closer to Moses until she achieved a position of laying side by side with him. Miss Kitty taught me a lesson in patience I have not forgotten and have indeed embraced.

Write Your Story

Most would agree that impatience has caused some degree of adversity in their lives, either as the result their overt actions or by the internal effects on their health. This may be just the time to pump up your patience muscles. Do not worry about opportunity, it will inevitable present itself as long as you have a goal and any kind of limit on your time or energy. At the gym of Patience Strength Training, injury is avoided by starting small and working your way up. It is also important to get adequate rest and nutrition to support the process. Warm up first by starting your day with a quiet time and taking your gratitude vitamins. The risk of injury is increased with haste, so allow ample time to complete each exercise. Start with a stretch by smiling and nodding at the elderly lady who, by fumbling in her purse, is slowing down the grocery line. Work the arms by waving ahead the driver who tied with you at the four way intersection, remembering to deep breathe between each set. With time and repetition, you will notice hypertrophy of your patience muscles, signaling a readiness to ramp up your work out. A driver may, for example, cut you off in traffic while simultaneously giving you a hand signal. In your mind, quietly thank him for providing you with a great opportunity to increase strength. Take a deep breath, review your goals and schedule, and adjust your mindset. As you smile and wave in the the driver's rear view mirror, your patience muscle contracts and expands. Feel the burn. You would have succeeded in staving off the negative effects of anger and, as a bonus, you would have confused and disappointed the offender at the very least. Do not be discouraged if some patience work outs are under par with your current level. It's about progress, not perfection and exercising patience is a reward in itself.

IDENTITY

What Science Says

"TO KNOW THYSELF IS THE BEGINNING OF wisdom."[259] This famous quote is often attributed to Socrates. Though the question of "who am I," is somewhat fluid throughout one's life, the quandary of identity is typically and most significantly worked through during adolescence. Identity is defined as who I am, the way I think about myself, the way I am viewed by the world, and the characteristics that define me. Psychologist Erik Erikson expands on this definition in adding that, an adolescent's main question is not only "Who am I?" but "Who do I want to be?"[260] "In addition

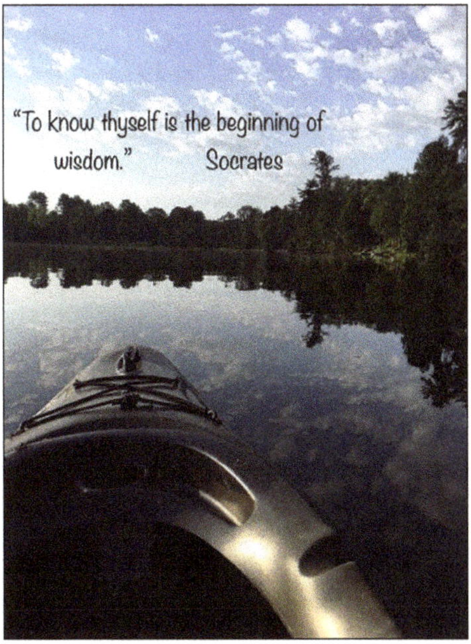

to carving out a personal identity based on the need for uniqueness, adolescents also acquire a social identity based on their membership in various groups; familial, ethnic, occupational, and others. "These group identities, in addition to satisfying the need for affiliation, help them define themselves in the eyes of both others and themselves."[261] (Althea E. Young PhD). Ultimately, teens want to create a sense of self that is consistent, meaning that they feel harmonious and in alignment in all areas. This is done by exploring options and "trying on various hats." Knowledge of one's identity is imperative because of its influence on confidence and security. Identity makes decision making easier by giving teens standards by which to make them. Parents, extended family, and teachers can facilitate the identity formation process by providing an understanding sounding board in a setting of unconditional love and acceptance. Teens are wise to listen to people who know them completely in developing their identity since how they define and describe themselves, ultimately controls their decisions and their behavior. An "identity crisis," or a questioning of one's identity may occur at any time in one's life when one is faced with a major challenge to their identity. Adjustments or major changes may occur at that time. Once one's identity is developed, regardless of age, it is healthy to keep exploring and reevaluating one's values, roles, and sense of self.

What God Says

A Christian's identity is inherent in their decision to be a follower of Christ. Since God created us **"in his own image,"** we are encouraged to learn how to be like Christ through studying the Bible. **"God created man in his own image, in the image of God he created him; male and female he created them."**[262] **(Genesis 1:27)** Followers of Christ should be able to be recognized by their virtues of self-discipline, faithfulness, obedience, charity, forgiveness, humility, and wisdom. In addition, when guidance in decision making is needed on matters, large or small, the Holy Spirit is available to Christ followers. Having access to well defined biblical commands and principals, along with the additional council of the Holy Spirit, makes a Christian's identity more likely to be consistent, harmonious and in alignment in all areas.

One of My Stories

As a child, I was called many things, depending on whose jurisdiction I was under and also the alcohol titer of my caretaker. This, I believe, made it challenging, at best, to build a consistent identity. I was called names such as "witch," one moment, to "beautiful movie star," the next. I was praised for A's on report cards then ridiculed and laughed at for misspeaking. Not having established a strong identity by which to base decisions early on resulted in an "identity crisis" in my thirties. This caused me to make some very poor and very disruptive decisions. It was not until

I accepted Jesus' offer of forgiveness much later and started learning about His character through reading the Bible, that I made the decision to identify with Him. Though I continue to be bombarded with secular values thru the media and much of society, the qualities I find in the Bible, self-discipline, faithfulness, obedience, charity, forgiveness, humility, and wisdom have proven worthy of emulating and strengthening and do provide a strong basis for making life decisions and for providing inner peace.

Write Your Story

How would you define yourself? If you're unsure, you might start by writing down your perccived values. The next step would be to talk to yourself as you go through your day making decisions. Say, for example, a good friend asks you to bring them on an errand in a car during a time when a social distancing mandate is in place, such as during a disease epidemic. You know that this violates the government's medical mandate but, at the same time, you do not want to disappoint your friend or have them think less of you. At this point, you may feel very uncomfortable and you may wish you could just avoid the situation. This is one of those opportunities for you to become aware of your values, and to be true to them, or in some cases, to adjust them. If abiding by rules and protecting the welfare of others are values that are important to you, you would tell your friend "no" in as nice a way as possible and be willing to accept the consequences. Your identity would be intact and your values would be reinforced. As you continue through your days, and question your rationale for deciding to proceed in one direction or another, you will discover what your real values are and you will be more likely to weigh future decisions against them. Increased inner peace and less stress results when your decisions and values align across all areas of your life. A bit of discomfort occurs when your values butt up against an unpopular decision, but it does get easier with time and the strengthened identity you develop is well worth it.

Creativity

What Science Says

Color outside the lines. Be messy. Feel the textures. Smell the smells. Take it all in. Children's innate creativity will grow and blossom if it is not contained in a box. If unstifled, creative children become creative adults and creativity paints a most positive picture of health.

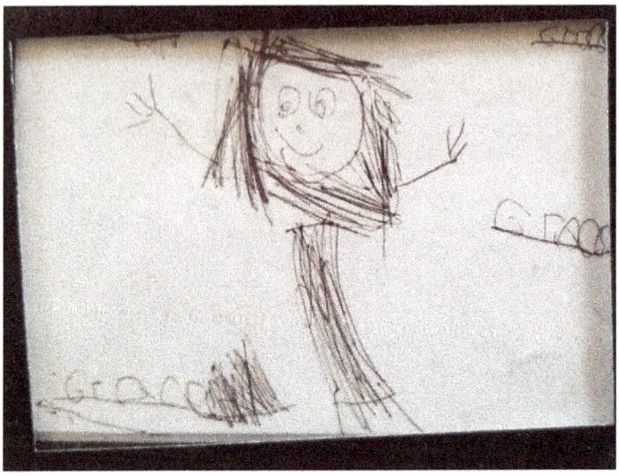

"Engaging in creative activities contributes to an "upward spiral" of positive emotions, and psychological well-being"[263] according to a recent New Zealand Study. The American Journal of Public Health finds that "creativity affects the brain and body leading to benefits like increased mood, decreased anxiety, heightened cognitive function, reduced risk of chronic illnesses and improved immune health. Creating artwork can also improve fine motor skills through small, purposeful movements, which may help to prevent pain and stiffness."[264] Researchers say that "creative pursuits work by building connections in the brain to strengthen cognitive reserve, or brain resilience, and subsequently preventing memory loss."[265] For those who have trouble expressing themselves, creating a visual representation of thoughts and feelings can be a simpler way to communicate thus reducing feelings of loneliness and isolation. Creativity is a unique health practice in that it provides pleasure and benefit before, during, and after it is done.

What God Says

The very first recorded act of God was to create. **"In the beginning God created the heavens and the earth."[266] (Genesis 1).** Since God then created us in his image, we are, by His design, creative beings. **"So God created mankind in his own image, in the image of God he created them; male and female he created them."[267] (Genesis 1:27)**. To live the best life possible, we are instructed to cultivate and use the creative gifts we've been given and, further, to do it with gusto. **"Do not neglect the gift you have, which was given you by prophecy when the council of elders laid their hands on you. Practice these things, immerse yourself in them, so that all may see your progress."[268] (First Timothy 4:14-15) "Whatever you do, do your work heartily, as for the Lord rather than unto men."[269] (Colossians 3:23)** I hear God saying to us, "work hard and have fun at creating in my style, all options open, including coloring outside the lines."

One of My Stories

According to Ursula Leguin, a noted speculative fiction author, "The creative adult is the child who survived."[270] This premise rings true to me it that, in facing various childhood experiences, I learned the prudence of paying very close attention to people and circumstances around me in order to strategically plan my actions. I also learned the fine art of day dreaming, a skill that allowed me to retreat to a finer place and time as needed. I was, in fact, dubbed by my teachers, the day dream queen of the fourth grade. Having been given generous latitude in self direction, eliminated many of the usual barriers to creativity. Since, in my family of origin, the model for "normal" was ill defined, my ability to "think outside the box" was never lost; it was in fact enhanced. Being challenged beyond my years by responsibility, required me to hone my creative talents. I enjoyed fancying myself a lady "MacGyver" when presented with seemingly unsolvable problems. Even now, my idea of a good time is repurposing a wounded toboggan into a decorative wall hanging, stenciling drab stair risers, or using rejected jewelry to glittify a lamp shade. Words are my creative tools for sharing my thoughts and emotions. Color, texture, shape, and design allow me to create peaceful and healing spaces. I am grateful for the circumstances that fueled my creativity and continues to expand and to express my worldly and my non worldly perspectives.

Write Your Story

What if the question were not "can I do it" but instead, how will I get this done"? What if, instead of painting the entire inside of your house beige, you select your colors for at least one room, around something you love love love, an "inspiration piece," like a favorite painting? One more "what if." What if you find yourself happy and excited whenever you present a dish you cooked like a work of art? Pop goes the weasel! You're jumped out of the box. Now close the lid so you don't climb back in. Life is your canvas. Don your smock and beret and create for happiness and health. The Creator is cheering you on.

Joy

What Science Says

"Joy is not in things; it is in us."[271] (Richard Wagner, composer) That joy is one of the positive qualities that enhances our health by boosting our immune systems, mediating stress and pain, and even increasing longevity is supported by multiple studies. Joy is akin to happiness but is much more substantial; it is not based upon current happenings or whether things are going well or not. According to Merriam-Webster Dictionary, "happiness is a state of well-being and contentment," primarily self-focused and rooted in the material world while joy is much deeper; it is derived from soul satisfying, emotional wellbeing."[272] Author J.D. Salinger gives us an apt analogy, "The most singular difference between happiness and joy is that happiness is a solid and joy is a liquid."[273] Since Joy is the prize, how do we acquire it? According to a 2019 UK study, "for us to be joyful we must not only discover but also follow our purpose and passion in life." Not surprisingly, having faith doubles the odds of achieving joy. "Faith and the acknowledgement that there is more going on than meets the eye creates peace of mind and letting go, and further, the study shows, that those without any spiritual grounding are twice as likely to be "very unhappy."[274] Achieving periods of happiness is easy. A job promotion, a phone call from a desirable person, a hot fudge sundae; are all happiness provoking. Previous chapters on the topics of service, social support, gratitude, and presence, are all steps towards enjoying happiness. When these same practices that produce happiness align with our values and passions, eureka; we have joy.

What God Says

Joy is a gift; it is one of the fruits of the spirit which results from having the indwelling of the Holy Spirit. This happens after we accept Jesus's gift of forgiveness for our sins and salvation. All of God's children have spiritual gifts; which might include things like wisdom, administration, hospitality, or healing. **"God has given each of us each a gift from his great variety of spiritual gifts. Use them well to serve one another."[275] (1 Peter 4:10)** The secret to real joy is being willing to use our gifts by allowing God to direct us in serving others. This also has the desirable effect of strengthening our relationship with God. **"I am full of joy because of the experience of knowing Jesus, and I want to invite you to share in that joy!"[276] (1John 1-4)** "To find real joy, you must shift from an inward focus—"It's all about me"—to an outward focus—"It's all about God and serving others."[277] (Rick Warren) Joy results from putting our trust in God, not in ourselves. **"Oh, the joys of those who trust the Lord."[278] (Psalm 40:4)**

One of My Stories

I wish I had had, as a young person, the prerogative of being concerned with the achievement of genuine joy alongside some worldly happiness but that is not my story. I dealt, instead, with the depression characteristic of the oldest of five children in an alcoholic family. I held the rank of "family hero," described in textbooks as "one who can identify other's needs and meet them, but is without an understanding of their own needs. As described, I felt "like a fraud and was subject to depressions which I hid from those around me."[279] The God I learned about in childhood catechism class was more judgmental than loving and I was fearful of both authority and other people's anger. Always in defensive mode, I learned to be excellent at control and found it safest to trust no one but myself. On the up side, while living my "family hero" role, I did learn to work hard, to persevere, and to be fiercely independent. I was headed down the road of alcoholism but was averted. Whether by my sweet grandmother's prayers or the promptings of the Holy Spirit, a desire was placed in my heart. I prayed for faith in God and He gave it to me. With my brother John, I accepted Jesus' gift of forgiveness of my sins and did an about face. Over the years I have grown

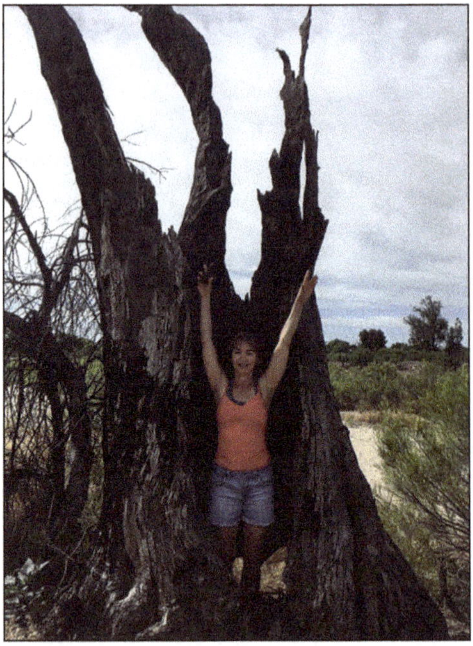

closer to God through studying the Bible, through obedience and through trusting Him more all the time. I now have a Father in God who loves me unconditionally and who I know in my heart is completely trustworthy. God leads me to use my spiritual gifts to serve. The true joy I now have continues to increase as I come to know and trust God more and find that, as promised, my joy withstands adversity and even grows through it.

Write Your Story

Happiness is a very good thing. Thinking positive thoughts, expressing gratitude, surrounding yourself with happy people; all good. You, like me, are one way ticket holders to this life so why not go for the gold; joy. You could start by deciding what activities do you love, love, love to do? Next, from the imaginary vantage point of sitting on the edge of your coffin, and looking back over your life, what about the world would you like to have had a positive effect on. Now combine these answers and get up. There is still time. What if, for example, you are gifted in singing and you would like to have had an effect on making people happier and more peaceful. Consider the other values and responsibilities you might have such as supporting a family and then search for opportunity. Your path to joy may be a full time job, an avocation or it may start with volunteer work. Once you combine your passions with your values you will have "found a job you enjoy doing, and you will never have to work again a day in your life."[280] (Mark Twain) If you have Jesus in your life, power up and ask (pray) for his direction. If not, consider inviting him in. If you are not ready, good news; God listens to all requests including a desire for "readiness." If you're still reluctant, be assured that God loves you and patiently waits. What might seem impossible, with God, is possible and, when it requires "endurance" and "faith," it will result in an even higher level of joy.

Gratitude

What Science Says

Thank you. I appreciate that. That was so nice of you. You know that the recipient of these expressions of gratitude feels a pleasant boost but, whoa, such gestures also back fire making us feel better as well. Gratitude can stand alone or it can precipitate or complement other health practices such as kindness and forgiveness. Willie Nelson went so far as to say, "When I started counting my blessings, my whole life turned around."[281] Science support's the positive health effects of gratitude in demonstrating that people who practice gratitude through interaction or even through journaling, enjoy a higher level of physical, psychological, and social health. Whether the finding that grateful people tend to exercise more and engage in other positive lifestyle practices or whether gratitude independently positively effects good health indicators, it really doesn't matter. The statistics are in as far as correlating gratitude with better health; stronger immune systems, less feelings of loneliness, better sleep, and more energy. Studies out of the the Greater Good Science Center at U.C. Berkeley suggest that "there may be a link between religion and gratitude citing a trial in which one group who were assigned to pray for their marital partner for four weeks felt much more gratitude towards their partner than the group who were assigned to just think positive thoughts about their partners."[282] In a culture of time restraints, praying appears to be the more efficient means of increasing gratitude and, in turn, health.

What God Says

The Bible is all about gratitude. **"Do not be anxious about anything, but in every situation, by prayer and petition, with thanksgiving, present your requests to God. And the peace of God, which transcends all understanding, will guard your hearts and your minds in Christ Jesus."[283] (Philippians 4:6-7) "Rejoice always, pray continually, give thanks IN all circumstances; for this is God's will for you in Christ Jesus."[284] (1 Thessalonians 5:16-18**. As with all instruction from God through scripture, God is directing us to the best path to follow. I will point out to you what it took me a decade to notice. I noticed that I am to give thanks IN all circumstances not FOR all circumstances. This means I don't have to be thankful for the fender bender I was in, for example, but I can look for something IN the situation to be grateful for; bumping into a long lost friend perhaps.

One of My Stories

I was pleasantly tired after a hike in the mountains with my grandkids. Pulling into my little lakeside cabin, I looked forward to doing a little sprucing up with fresh cut flowers and a change of linens in preparation for my sister's visit. I was greeted by a downed hibiscus tree in the front yard and a broken couch inside. My mom was waiting for me to visit at the nursing home and my sister texted from midflight to ask me to shop for a few items she would like to have in the cabin for her visit. An attitude of gratitude was a cake walk while hiking the Adirondacks with my grandkids but my initial reaction to my current situation was anything but gracious. I allowed myself to wallow in self-pity and despair until the all too familiar uncomfortable feeling welling up inside prompted me to offer up a prayer, "God, help. I'm writing about gratitude here, God". I had the impression he was telling me, "Here's a practice opportunity for you, my daughter." "Thank you God", I offered up. The gratitude ice was broken. From there it wasn't much of a leap to thank the couch sales people for their assistance in purchasing the ideal new couch, and to thank God for giving me the strength and the tools to clean up the tree situation. I then felt moved to express a grand finale burst of thank you's for the time I would soon get to spend with my sister, a tidy yard, and an anticipated super pretty living room. I could have saved myself a lot of turmoil had I gone directly to looking for the things to be thankful

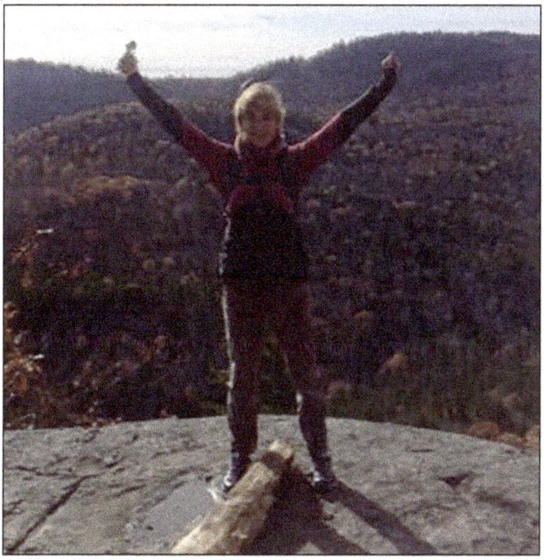

for IN the circumstance. I am especially grateful that God isn't done with me yet.

Write Your Story

Since thankful words and actions can be doled out from a virtual unlimited supply and are proven to enhance your health, why not offer appreciation at every opportunity? After you experience the benefits of a more grateful heart, ready yourself for the ultimate gratitude challenge? At the onset of the next adverse event, and you know it will occur, find a thing or two in the situation to be grateful for then go ahead, say it. "Even though I got a flat tire," for example, if I didn't, I would not have experienced the satisfaction of having successfully changed a tire. Admittedly this radical proclamation of gratitude is never our default response but, if consistently practiced, I can attest that the payback is profound.

Surrender

What Science Says

"Let it go. Let it go." Not only a popular hit song but also a healthy way to live. Trying to single handedly run the show is exhausting and it makes us sick and unhappy. Why then do we do it? "We try to manage other people and circumstances so we won't feel hurt, nervous, stressed, disappointed or worried,"[285] concludes Dr. Michael Kragt, a licensed psychologist at Grace Counseling in Denver. We can, however, make a decision to surrender those things we are not responsible for or are unable to change. Surrender is defined as "complete acceptance of what is plus sufficient faith that all will be well, even without our input."[286] The Twelve Steps of Alcoholics Anonymous is a prime example of the effects of surrender on recovery from a heretofore incurable disease, alcoholism. The third of the twelve steps of Alcoholics Anonymous, "Made a decision to turn our wills and our lives over to the care of God as we understood him,"[287] is critical to success in achieving sobriety, with the only required action being that of "willingness." Faith cannot be minimized as key to surrender but faith does not necessarily require a belief in God. "Faith can simply be the belief that we will benefit from even negative experiences. This benefit may be personal growth, a life lesson, or a nudge in the right direction by our unconscious."[288] (Psychology Today). "If our surrender is to God," according to a Mayo Clinic Study, "outcomes tend to be associated with lower reported stress and therefore putting us at lowered risk for stress-related health problems."[289] "Some people believe holding on and hanging in there are signs of great strength. However, there are times when it takes much more strength to know when to let go and then do it."[290] (Ann Landers)

What God Says

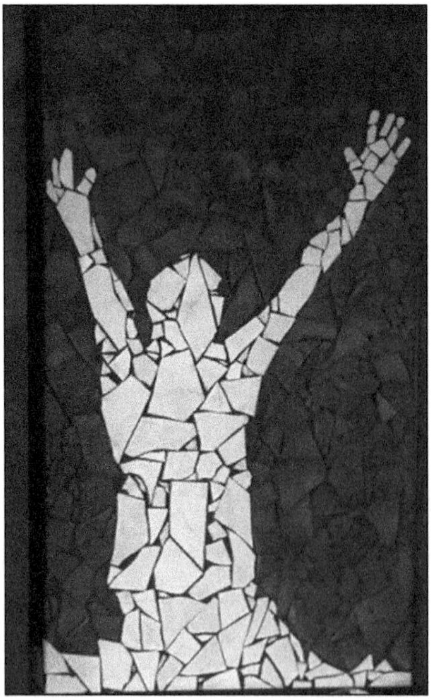

God consistently invites us to surrender our problems to him, **"Cast all your anxiety on Him because he cares for you."[291] (1 Peter 5:7) "The righteous cry out, and the Lord hears them; he delivers them from all their troubles."[292] (Psalm 34:17)** After suffering on the cross for us, Jesus performed the ultimate act in the surrender of his spirit, **"Then Jesus**

cried out again with a loud voice and gave up his spirit."[293] (Matthew 27:50) Cited as Jesus response to his disciples on how to pray, the "Our Father" is a prayer of promise, faith and surrender, **"Our Father in heaven, hallowed be your name. Your kingdom come, your will be done, on earth as it is in heaven. Give us this day our daily bread, and forgive us our debts, as we also have forgiven our debtors. And lead us not into temptation, but deliver us from evil."[294] (Matthew 6:9-13)** Amen.

One of My Stories

Neither politics, parenting nor people have posed the primary impediments in my life. Self-will, along with my perceived need to control, have often caused great havoc in my life. Having fancied myself head of household in an out of control alcoholic home, attempting to manage the chaos seemed to be the wise approach. After my graduation into the real world, husbands, employees, family and friends retaliated against my efforts to micro manage their lives though, in my eyes, I was saving them from themselves. Five marriages, four degrees and ten jobs later, I have surrendered my crown to an omnipresent, omnipotent, omniscient and loving God. This decision has given me a life of freedom, peace, and health. I start my day with a prayer I borrowed from Alcoholics Anonymous, the Third Step Prayer, "God, I offer myself to Thee – to build with me and to do with me as Thou wilt. Relieve me of the bondage of self, that I may better do Thy will. Take away my difficulties, that victory over them may bear witness to those I would help of Thy Power, Thy Love, and Thy Way of Life. May I do Thy will always!"[295] When my conscience pokes me to let me know I'm trying to grab back the reins, I send up a eloquent prayer, "help," and He gets me back on track.

Write Your Story

Sometimes management and control are outlined in your employee job description or are integral to your responsibilities as a parent. Within your designated role, you do have some latitude as to how you choose to manage. At home, the degree of control of your children required for their safety and guidance can be done with love and with some flexibility. You might choose to manage morning wake up with, "Would you like me to wake you up for school or would you like to set your own alarm clock?" for example. At work, you might sit down with a habitually tardy employee and demonstrate caring management by making it well defined what is expected and clearly putting the responsibility for the consequences of their behavior in their control. In the areas of your life where you are not the designated boss, you might consider taking back your freedom, accepting the things you cannot change and practicing going with the flow. "How important is it?" is a great tool by which to measure whether situations even warrant an energy expenditure. Managing through manipulation and intimidation is ineffective and unhealthy for all involved, while surrendering control is life giving. Most importantly, giving up trying to control the future, allows you to fully be in the present. It is said so well by Eckhart Tolle “Always say ‘yes’ to the present moment. Surrender to what is. “Say ‘yes’ to life–and see how life starts suddenly to start working for you rather than against you.”[296]

Work

What Science Says

Is work good for your health or bad for your health. The answer is a resounding yes to both options. Aside from the obvious need for food, shelter, and designer jeans, studies show that "work is generally good for your health. As well as providing a financial reward, our job gives many of us self-esteem, companionship and status. There is good evidence that being out of work is bad for your health. Laid-off workers are far more likely than those continuously employed workers to have fair or poor health, and to develop a stress-related condition, such as stroke, heart attack, heart disease, or arthritis. Unemployed Americans are far more likely than employed Americans to be diagnosed with depression and to report feelings of sadness and worry."[297] (Robert Wood Johnson Foundation Publication March 2013.) Too much work can be detrimental to our health but how much is too much? "Results shows that the average worker is at the office about 47 hours a week, but a person's mental health begins to take a nose dive after working for 39 hours in any given week. At the same time, people who worked very little also had worse mental health — the same as people who worked way too much."[298] (Social Science & Medicine). Working conditions and work status also impacts the effects of work on our health. The studies found that "those in higher status roles were less likely to die of heart disease than those in lower status roles.

It is thought those in higher status roles are able to make meaningful decisions in their work and have a greater level of control in their life. As we would expect, job satisfaction greatly affects our health. A large scale meta-analysis of almost 500 studies has provided a clear indication of the immensely strong relationship between job satisfaction and both mental and physical health."[299] (E B Faragher, M Cass, C L Cooper.) Summarily, the recipe for healthful work includes, choosing work that we enjoy doing, using tools that allow us to effectively do our work, and carving out a reasonable schedule in safe, comfortable conditions.

What God Says

God himself modeled the perfect work formula in creating the universe; work for six days at something you love, stand back to assure that your work is good, then take an entire day to rest. He rewarded newly created Adam and Eve in the Garden of Eden with the gift of work. **"Be fruitful and increase in number; fill the earth and subdue it. Rule over the fish... the birds... and over every living creature that moves on the ground."[300] (Genesis 1:28).** We are instructed that we all should work if possible, **"Everyone should work if they're able to. The one who is unwilling to work shall not eat."[301] (2 Thessalonians 3:10)** In our jobs, we are to be respectful of those we report to while keeping in mind that we ultimately report to the highest Authority, God, who loves us and is always just. **"Whatever you do, work at it with all your heart, as working for the Lord, not for men, since**

you know that you will receive an inheritance from the Lord as a reward. It is the Lord Christ you are serving."[302] (Colossians 3:23) As a strong backup, God is a Consultant we can call on anytime during the day if we find ourselves slipping into a place of insecurity or self-doubt about our job. **"If any of you lacks wisdom, you should ask God, who gives generously to all without finding fault, and it will be given to you."[303] (James 1:5)**

One of My Stories

My resume includes a variety of jobs compiled over a sixty year span. A sampling includes child care, ice cream server, waitress, secretary, clerk, registered nurse, aerobics instructor, nurse practitioner, author, as well multiple volunteer jobs and, most importantly, mom, grandmother, and wife. Finding wisdom in the Bible and talking with other believers, is finally bringing me to the brink of discovering my healthy

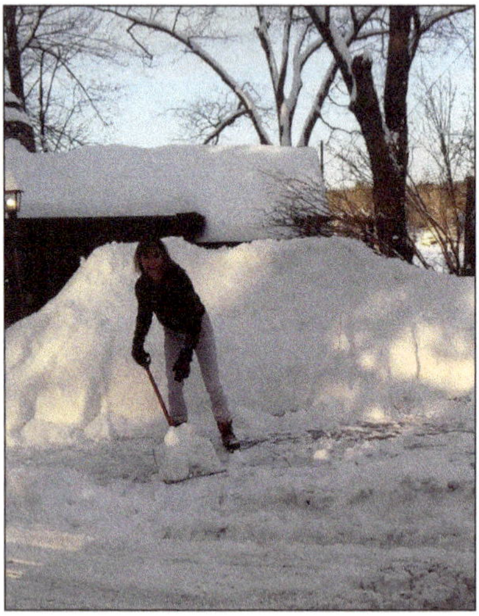

work formula. I've learned what it is like to work too many hours at too many jobs while trying to juggle school and family. I've experienced having life zooming by like a nonstop train sans sleeper car, moving much too fast to appreciate the view much less to stop to participate in it. Though always open for improvement, healthy work for me has evolved to this pretty simple three step process; 1. Setting and recording my life goals and making important decisions based on these goals. 2. Getting up very early, to read the Bible then being quiet to "hear" direction as to how I might apply what I've read to my life. 3. Adhering to a principle found in "Experiencing God," by Henry Blackaby; each morning taking the time to observe what God is doing around me, and asking Him how I might contribute to His plan. Currently this process is allowing me a schedule to work at the things I love; writing and one on one ministry. This still leaves me time to spend with family, to maintain a little respite cabin, and to take care of my personal health. I continue to search for the word "retirement" in the Bible.

Write Your Story

In my work, I've been privileged to see lives change radically for the better and health improve when someone I've come to know makes the necessary changes to match their passions and skills with their work. Admittedly, such a change usually does not happen overnight. For you, once you define your dream job goal, you are then ready to draft a plan, a budget, and a time line to achieve your goal, keeping in mind, job satisfaction, work hours, environment, compensation, and contribution to others. When obstacles emerge, go to plan B, or go around or through. Work is good; best when it matches your uniqueness. Go for it. Your dream job awaits.

Hospitality

What Science Says

Tea time. Hospitality is a warm and nurturing blend of the finest of teas; kindness, generosity, and social connectedness. Indulged in separately, each individual ingredient has proven to enhance the health and the happiness of both the server and the recipient while the infusion of the three is shown to be synergistically beneficial. Motel Eight is not the first place to beckon the weary traveler with the promise to "leave the light on". The roots of hospitality are ancient, initially viewed as a mandate from the "Gods" established to protect the sojourner as well as the resident. The implication was, "if you take care of me, then I won't hurt you". Carrying the hospitality concept forward to today, we cannot help but notice that industries, such as healthcare, have learned that providing a service in a hospitable manner is very good for business. On a broad scale, or in our individual homes, three elements; a warm welcome, a meeting of needs, and personal interaction are the keys to hospitality. Once a stranger, a client, or a friend is securely within the arms of hospitality, interactions can be enjoyed and benefited from. Drink to health and happiness the fine tea of hospitality.

What God Says

The Bible is abundantly clear regarding hospitality with God's two greatest commandments being "to love God and love others." **Leviticus 19:34** says, **"You shall treat the stranger that sojourns with you as the native among you, and you shall love him as yourself."**[304] Jesus later tells us in **Matthew 25:40** that **"whatever we do for the least of people, we do for him"** later adding, **"Do not neglect to show hospitality to strangers, for thereby some have entertained angels unaware."**[305] **(Hebrews 13:2)** The famous story of the Good Samaritan points out that we are to be so radical as to show hospitality even to those who are perceived as our enemies. Those who do step out in faith through Ministries such as Habitat for Humanity, Samaritan's Purse, and Doctors Without Borders, are more than happy to expound on the effects of answering the call to hospitality on their own lives. Opportunity to provide hospitality is limitless in scope, and time. Again, God's commands, though often conflicted with worldly norms, are always in the best interest of our long term health and happiness.

One of My Stories

The childhood memory of the aroma of freshly baked bread, the simmering of marinara sauce and the sight of my Grandma Gug's broad smile and open arms still brings a smile to my face and a warming to my heart. It was the good fortune of my entire family, that my sister Tisha inherited our Grandma Gug's gift of hospitality. Tisha, or "Aunt TT," as displayed on her Arizona license plate, has made herself and her home a place of refuge and healing to all of us; be it parent, sibling, nieces and nephews, or friends. After following our airline flight across the country last April, Tisha

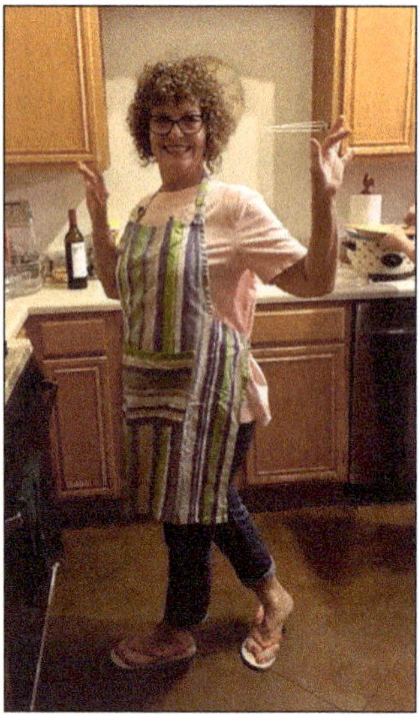

promptly met us at the Tucson airport open armed and smiley faced with water bottle in hand. We started our conversation right where we left off six months prior. I walked in her front door and right out the back to the patio. I fully exhaled as I melted into her chaise, strategically placed in the Arizona sun, surrounded by freshly arranged flowers. I gave absolutely no thought about whether I had committed a social faux pas in my haste because I knew that Tisha loved me no matter what. We laughed. We talked. We ate. We walked. It was, as always, hospitality at its finest. I would consider myself to be her favorite person in the entire world if I did not know that, whether it's by air or by sea, whether alone or with an entire family, everyone Tisha graces with her hospitality, is similarly blessed and, of course, so is Tisha.

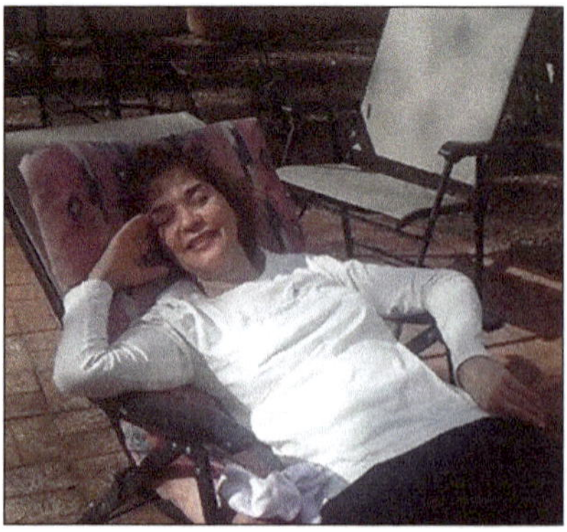

Write Your Story

Knowing that all aspects of hospitality, kindness, generosity, and social connectedness are good for the health and welfare of all concerned, how might you effect a life change or two, short of inviting the entire neighborhood to dinner twice a week? You and the people you choose to host will benefit from your hospitality to whatever degree or in whatever venue you choose to provide it. A bed offered to a fellow employee during an ice storm, a coffee and a chit chat with a grieving friend or the offer to play with a toddler or two for a few hours while their parents go on a date are just a few of the many rewarding options your might choose from to practice your hospitality. Now imagine volunteering at an Open Door Mission so you could regularly eat, sit and talk with guests? How might these conversations comfort and grow both of you? As you are enjoying your hospitality role, always keep in mind, you may "be entertaining angels unaware."

Humility

What Science Says

The poet Alfred Tennyson is noted to have written that "humility is the highest virtue, the mother of them all."[306] Another great thinker C.S. Lewis writes, "To be humble is not to think less of oneself, but to think of oneself less."[307] Humility is defined by Merriam-Webster as "the freedom from pride or arrogance."[308] The virtue of humility can greatly affect our health. In order to be poised for assimilating health knowledge into actual life change, we must be humble enough to believe there is indeed a need in us for such change. On the care side of the equation, a humble practitioner realizes that "nobody cares how much they know until those people know how much they're cared for."[309] (Rick Pitino). An effective provider/patient scenario could look something like this: The health provider prescribes weight loss as a treatment for knee pain. The provider then respectfully interacts with the patient to tailor the treatment to the patient's personal preferences and abilities. The patient, in turn, accepts the provider's recommendation as an opportunity to improve his health, feeling free to engage in an interchange with the provider until a plan is mutually agreed upon.

What God Says

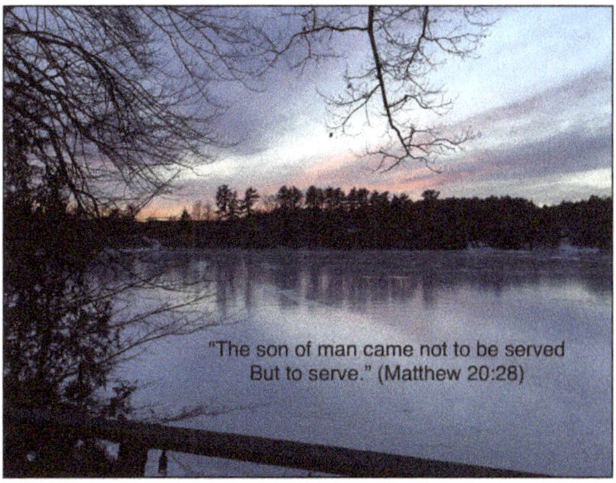

Jesus was the ultimate model of humility during his earthly ministry. "**For even the Son of Man did not come to be served, but to serve, and to give his life as a ransom for many."[310] (Matthew 20:28)** The Bible is clear on God's view on humility and, it's counter, pride. "**God opposes the proud, but gives grace to the humble."[311] (James 4:6) "Do nothing from rivalry or conceit, but in humility count others more significant than yourselves. Let each of you look not only to his own interests, but also to the interests of others."[312] (Philippians 2:3-5)** Jesus lived humility, teaching us through his actions and through his Word to humbly follow Him on the humility path to abundance and health.

One of My Stories

"You should be proud," I was told after scoring an A on my vocabulary quiz. This version of proud, meant receiving praise for having studied hard enough to produce a good test score. I later heard, "don't let your pride keep you from applying again for a head nurse position." I now recognize this version of "pride" to be an arrogant pride. I was mistakenly thinking that applying for a job I had been previously turned down for would require me to have to change the inflated, albeit shaky, image I had of myself. Today, whether I get a job or not, I thank God, not myself, knowing that He will work it for the good in the long run. It takes tremendous pressure off me knowing that it's not just about me and that I am never alone. I have learned from the great thinkers, Tennyson, Lewis and, the greatest of all, Jesus. As I humbly give God the glory, He lightens my load and gives me peace and health.

Write Your Story

The world tells you, "You're entitled to behave however you like and still enjoy the good health and happiness you desire." If this mindset is not producing the results you would like, let me present another approach. First, let us look at one health behavior, diet, objectively. If you choose to consume one third more calories than your body requires, you will eventually become obese, putting you at twenty times the risk of someday developing knee pathology and the resultant pain. You would eventually require knee replacement surgery. It's not about ideology or political correctness. It is simple math. Replacing the illogical "entitlement" approach with a humble willingness to learn, gives you the power to make smarter health choices. If you continue in the open to learn mode, you will inevitably discover that taking the focus off yourself through helping others produces the greatest health and happiness. You could test it out in a way that suits your talents and preferences. It can be as simple as picking up the meal ticket for a uniformed soldier in a restaurant to as complex as building homes for Habitat for Humanity. Ironically you will find that the way to make yourself happy, is to redirect your focus away from yourself and direct it towards serving others.

INTEGRITY

What Science Says

"WHAT YOU SEE IS WHAT YOU GET," IS what can be said of a person with integrity. Integrity is defined as "doing the right thing at all times and in all circumstances, whether or not anyone is watching, and no matter what the consequences." A person of integrity acts the same no matter where they go and they are truthful in every area of their lives. Just as constructing one floor of a building out of soft pine and the others out of steel would compromise the building's structural integrity, so would being honest in most areas of one's life, while cheating in one area, such as their marriage, would compromise an individual's integrity. In other words, an imbalance in tensile strength would be as dangerous to the health of the building as an imbalance in personal integrity would be to one's personal health; erosive disease and ultimate collapse would inevitably ensue. A life lived with integrity is undeniably not an easy road to choose, but it is proven to be the most sought after quality in a leader, an employee, a friend or a partner. It is the most important success indicator of an individual, a group, or a nation. Having homogeneous integrity in all aspects of one's life, be it spiritual, professional, marital, or parental, makes for a durable person, able to better withstand the storms of life and far better able to be relied on by others.

What God Says

God blesses us when we live our lives with integrity. Jesus said in the Sermon on the Mount that **"you are blessed when your heart is pure."**[313] "A pure heart" today is synonymous with integrity. **(Matthew 5:8) Confession and repentance are the first steps to change to a life of integrity**, saying to God, "I was wrong. I accept your gift of dying on the cross as payment for my wrongs, and I plan on living with integrity from now on." We are told to have integrity in keeping promises. **"People who promise things they never give are like clouds and wind that bring no rain."**[314] **(Proverbs 25:14)** Persons of integrity say what they mean and mean what they say. The Bible offers a rock solid way to live a life of integrity. It is, like Jesus, **"the light and the truth."**

One of My Stories

When I consider people I've known who model integrity, my grandparents, Carmela and Salvatore Gugliotta, immediately come to mind. They held firm to high standards in every area of their lives. As a young couple bravely venturing from Sicily to realize the American dream, they strictly abided by American immigration rules, written and implied, diligently speaking English and not allowing their nine children to even learn Italian. They succeeded in assimilating into American culture so well that each of their four sons proudly served in the military, their daughters all becoming respected wives, moms, and professionals. Fiercely self-sufficient, my Grandparents raised their large family through the Depression by virtue of hard work; railroad employment, gardening, hunting, and sewing. In the spirit of self-sufficiency, my Grandfather, in one instance, may have overreacted a bit to a gesture of social support offered in the form of a food basket. The food basket was brought to their door with the assumption that they were a family in need. My proud grandfather turned the "hand out" bearer away with his shot gun. Carmela and Salvatore made decisions about their sixty year marriage, child rearing and community relations based on well ingrained standards, the Ten Commandments. My Grandmother lived her life by what she taught us that "if you treat

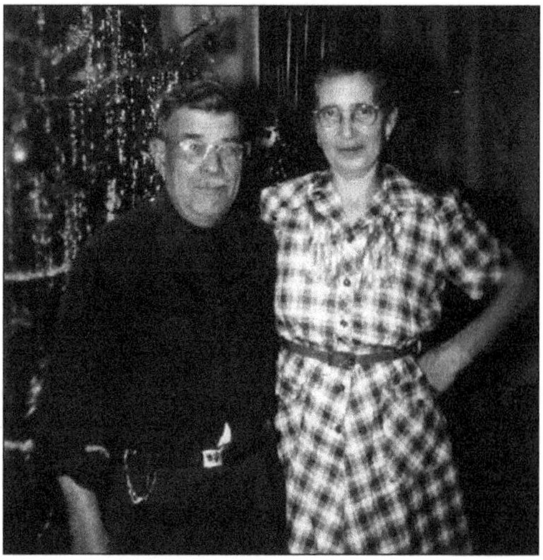

people with love, you will get love back." She was up every day before dawn to pray and to attend church. When, as grandchildren, we got to stay over, we regularly observed my Grandfather quietly praying over his vast garden. Integrity, manifested by consistency and fairness, made us, as Grandchildren, feel completely safe and loved whenever we were under their care. Leading by example, Grandma and Grandpa modeled integrity to nine children, over forty grandchildren and multiple other relatives and friends. Confucius aptly sums up the potential effects of their lives lived with integrity. "The strength of a nation derives from the integrity of the home."[315]

Write Your Story

Let's say you're not exactly walking crooked but you sense that you're somehow off balance. Your extremities are all functioning and aligned; physical integrity is intact. Your conscience, however, is making you feel uneasy so you look inward to your internal integrity. When you can give yourself some quiet time, you do a "play back" of the various areas of your life. You've been good to your spouse, even ran away from flirty Fran at work. Check. You tithed ten per at church with a happy heart. Check. You apologized to your son for over reacting. Check. You improved your score at computer solitaire at work. Buzzz! Even though you play solitaire much less than anyone else and you're never tardy for work, your conscience receptors convict you that you are stealing your employer's time. You then make a decision to fold your game. The more you allow your conscience to shape your behavior, the finer tuned it will become and the sooner the buzzer will sound. This may initially sound restrictive but, paradoxically, it is liberating. Your integrity will increase and you will reap the benefits; higher self-esteem, respect from others, success, and the positive influence on those around you. "Oh no. I'll never have any fun again," you may think. Ask anyone who has tried it both ways, including me. Integrity is more exciting, effective, energizing, and more excellent than deceit, especially in the, not too far off, long run. Tim Tebow, who is privileged with both fame and money says it well." My integrity means more to me than any fame or money. When I say something, I want people to take it to the bank that I mean it and believe in it."[316]

Routine

What Science Says

"Up in the mornin' and out to school. The teacher is teachin' the Golden Rule." Chuck Berry's lyrics to the "School Days" tune, in a whimsical, rhythmic way, describes a routine day in the life of a student. Children, as well as adults, benefit from having a routine to provide structure and discipline in their lives. Having a daily routine, contrary to what some might surmise, is found, not to decrease, but to actually increase, our freedom, our productivity, and our creativity. Routine also significantly lowers our stress levels. A daily routine allows us to build good habits, such as exercise, into our day and nudge out bad habits such as binging on television. Developing our own personal routine allows us to prioritize our activities in respect to our life goals, culling out the least relevant. Our efficiency is improved by appropriating activities to the time of day that best fit our personal rhythm. Writing or studying, for some people, for example, might be best scheduled in the quiet of the morning while shopping might be better to plan for late afternoon. Those of us with

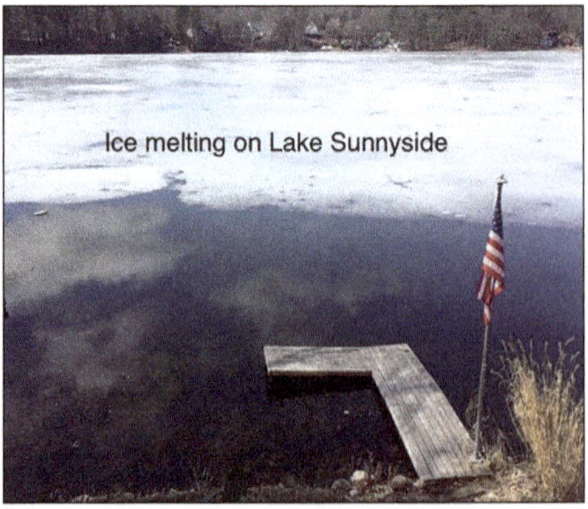
Ice melting on Lake Sunnyside

an established routine are able to reserve guilt free portions of our day to nap, to visit, or to do absolutely nothing. Our creativity is let loose because our minds are not bogged down with ongoing planning and recalibrating the balance of the day. Our self-esteem is boosted by having a daily routine, not only by being much more successful at meeting goals but also by way of consistently sticking to it. In times of the unplanned turmoil that life invariable presents, having a routine, reduces stress by evoking a sense of normalcy. Even watching nature effortlessly flow thru its routine of leaves falling, lake ice melting and birds migrating back gives us a sense of security during trying times. Needless to say, our routine is uniquely ours, met to be reviewed and refined by us as individuals, by time, by day, and by life season. If we want to have some control over our character development and our contribution to the world, it is wise to plan our own daily routine rather than have it happen to us, as, "We are what we repeatedly do."[317] (Aristotle)

What God Says

Jesus modeled healthy living by example. Scripture describes routines being practiced in both the old and the new testaments. **"Very early in the morning, while it was still dark, Jesus got up, left the house and went off to a solitary place, where he prayed"[318] (Mark 1:35)** The Israelites were told, **"Six days you shall labor and do all your work, but the seventh day is the Sabbath of the Lord your God. For in six days the Lord made the heavens and the earth, the sea**

and all that is in them, and rested the seventh day. Therefore the Lord blessed the Sabbath day and hallowed it."[319] (Exodus 20:8-11) Daniel, while living in threatening conditions and under the rule of an unpredictable ruler, held fast to his routine of praying three times a day, **"He got down on his knees three times a day and prayed and gave thanks before his God, as he had done previously."[320] (Daniel 6:10)** Proverbs, a book of the Bible replete with wise counsel, advocates for aspects of routine, diligence and careful planning in, **"The plans of the diligent lead to profit as surely as haste leads to poverty."[321] (Proverbs 21:5)**. It would be remiss not to mention the intricate routines by which God has created the universe to seamlessly function in harmony.

One of My Stories

As I write this post, we are in the midst of the Corona Virus Pandemic. I am grateful that, in this season of my life, living by a routine is well ingrained and I have had sufficient practice in resisting the urge to stray too far from it. In deciding what to fit into my routine, I reference my life goals; "love God and love each other through communicating truth and providing service". Early to bed and early to rise works well for me, starting my day with reading, meditating and writing. Next, is exercise, work and a power nap followed by communicating with family and friends. Evening is debriefing time with my husband and relaxing with social media and television viewing. We wind up the day with prayer. Sunday involves church, or, currently, telechurch, then some couch time. I consciously build "margin" into my routine in case God puts an unplanned service opportunity in my path. Without having had an established routine I would likely be frantically reacting to the hysteria being communicated by the media. I would be feeling stressed and would be much less productive. Observing God's established routines of the snow melting, and the sun's warmth increasing reassures me that this pandemic is but a blip in the bigger picture and life does go on. The Bible also reminds me that **"The earth is the LORD's, and everything in it, the world, and all who live in it; for he founded it on the seas and established it on the waters."[322] (Psalm 24:1-2)**

Write Your Story

If you do currently have a daily routine, you can attest to it's value, particularly in times of unrest. You might consider evaluating your routine at intervals to see if it needs to be tweaked to better suit your goals. Notice how you have been building your knowledge and your skills and accomplishing your goals by adhering to your routine. Give yourself kudos for this. If you do not have a routine or, if you or your family are temporarily displaced from your usual routine; good news. You can sit down right now, establish a daily routine and help each other stick to it. You might choose to see it as an excellent opportunity to bond, corroborate, and create a sense of normalcy and security for yourself and for others in your household. The effect of a routine on productivity and the mediation of stress will increase even more with time. If you are cruising along with your daily routine but have a gentle, yet persistent, sense that something important is missing, consider doing what I did, add spending time with God and see what happens.

Presence

What Science Says

"Do not dwell in the past, do not dream of the future, concentrate the mind on the present moment."[323] (Buddha). Concentrating on the present moment allows us to "savor" the experience we are in to the maximum, making it possible for us to reap the health and the happiness benefits that result from decreased stress. According to a Harvard University study, "people spend forty seven per cent of their waking hours thinking about something other than what they are doing."[324] "Mindfulness" is the process of purposely bringing one's attention to experiences occurring in the present moment without judgment. It is one method of training our minds to focus on the now. Being in the present precludes rumination about past "woulda, shoulda, coulda's"and worry about future "what if's." When we are able to "keep our heads where our feet are at," we are fully tuned in with all five of our senses. Staying in the present could make the experience of a children's choral recital a virtual banquet to the senses. We could choose to enjoy each unique little face, the sweet sounds of singing, the smell of spring air outside, the feel of wooden gym bleachers and the anticipated taste of bake sale treats. Alternately, we could elect to perceive the same experience as, "I feel so bad I was late for the last concert. I'll never forget how sad she looked. My, she does look so sweet singing with her friends. I wonder how much longer this is going to last. I probably won't get my work done tonight." Each scenario is equal in duration; the first a relaxing, healthful mix of sensations and emotions; the second, just a wasted passage of time. The good news is, we have a choice. "Yesterday is history, tomorrow is mystery, but today is a gift. That's why it is called present." We need only accept it.

What God Says

"God encourages his followers to "fear not" 365 times in the Bible, once for each day of the year,"[325] (Pastor Rick Warren) Scripture tells us that we have just the right amount to handle life one day without reaching backward or forward for more. "**Therefore do not be anxious about tomorrow, for tomorrow will be anxious for itself. Sufficient for the day is its own trouble."[326] (Matthew 6:34)** There is no merit in dwelling on mistakes we have made in the past. We need only accept Jesus' gift of forgiveness. **"If we confess our sins, He is faithful and just to forgive us our sins and to cleanse us from all unrighteousness."[327](1 John 1:98)** God, in his love for us, goes so far as to say that he does not even remember our sins once we have confessed and repented. So why should we remember them? **"For I will be merciful toward their iniquities, and I will remember their sins no more."[328] (Hebrews 8:12)** Allowing ourselves to be burdened by the past or to fret about the future is not what God desires for us, his children. He has given us his extraordinary creation to learn from and to enjoy. Keeping all of our intellect and senses tuned into the moment, while keeping just enough experience in mind to make smart decisions and just the right portion of planning in mind to do His will, enables us to live and to enjoy life to the extent God intended.

One of My Stories

If there were a Worry Award or an Over Thinkers Tournament, I would carry home trophies. I challenge myself at the start of each day, and throughout the day, to keep myself in the moment. Given free reign, my mind would rob me of fully enjoying experiences like taking a springtime walk around a lake. Instead of noticing the parallel slant of the sun on the violet hued grass, my mind would, instead, stew over a "shoulda" situation that occurred in the past. It could then use my well-developed imagination to "what if" a future concern. I am all about planning for the future and learning from past experiences but I've found that these very functional activities need not displace the serenity and the pleasure of intentionally living in the moment. Keeping myself focused on whatever experience is in front of me takes concerted effort on my part but the rewards are amazing and, to my surprise,

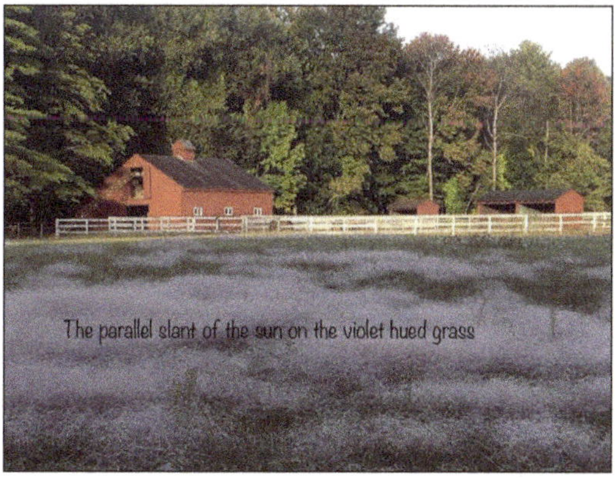
The parallel slant of the sun on the violet hued grass

I find I have never lost an opportunity by not allowing my mind to wander in either direction. As Mark Twain said, "I have known a great many troubles, but most of them never happened."[329]

Write Your Story

If you want to experience this one life you have been given to the nth degree, one big step in that direction would be to give yourself the gift of presence. You can start small and work your way up; like everything, perfection comes with practice. You might clear the stage of your mind by starting your day with some short and some long term planning. There. That is done. Now let go of it. Next, take a deep breath and intentionally down shift your gears. Walk slowly and move slowly. Slow is efficient. There is much less milk spilling, key losing, and dog escaping. Be mindful of your breakfast selection and preparation. Next comes the Pièce de résistance. Chew and savor the taste, texture, smell, and sight of each bite of your Cheerios and banana, Pop Tart, or Eggs Benedict. Smell the coffee. As you're chewing, look around the room for beauty; the sun nurturing a window plant or your child's face looking to you for a smile. Take another big breath. Be grateful. As for me, I say, "thank you God." For the balance of the day, remain vigilant. Look where your feet are and bring your mind back there. You are now in that moment. Realizing that life comes at you quickly sometimes and that some tasks require automatic, calculated, or data based responses, when opportunity does arise to "slow and know," tap softly on the brakes and indulge. It's your present if you choose to open it.

Sobriety

What Science Says

The entertainment, sports, and food industries have been remarkably successful in capitalizing on their annual investment of two billion dollars in advertisement to convince us that alcohol will make us happy, attractive, popular and affluent, and additionally, that it's even good for our health. A measurable indicator of their success is that excessive alcohol consumption, defined as greater than eight four ounce glasses of wine per week or more than three in one day for women, is now the third leading cause of preventable death in the United States. To compound its impact, alcohol also increases the magnitude of cause number one, smoking, and cause number two, obesity. Far less popular, and with much less funding for advertising, the Centers for Disease Control, the American Dietary Association and the American Heart Association make it clear that "no one should begin drinking alcohol or drink it more often on the basis of potential health benefits. Indeed, for some people, avoiding alcohol is the best course."[330] It is well demonstrated that drinking too much over time causes chronic physical and mental health issues. Heavy drinking can cause liver damage, cardiovascular disease, and multiple types of cancer. On the flip side, recent studies on the effects of trials of sobriety demonstrated that participants reported better sleep, weight loss, clearer thinking, and had measurably improved blood pressure readings and improved liver and glucose lab tests.

What God Says

Wine has been referenced and cautioned against in the Bible from the beginning. **"Wine is a mocker, and beer a brawler; whoever is led astray by them is not wise."[331] (Proverbs 20:1) "Be of sober spirit, be on the alert Your adversary, the devil, prowls around like a roaring lion, seeking someone to devour."[332] (1Peter5:8-9) "Let us behave properly as in the day, not in carousing and drunkenness, not in sexual promiscuity and sensuality, not in strife and jealousy."[333] (Romans 13:13) "And do not get drunk with wine, for that is dissipation, but be filled with the Spirit."[334](Ephesians 5:18) "It is not for kings to drink wine, nor for rulers to crave beer. For they will drink and forget what has been decreed, and deprive all the oppressed of their rights."[335] (Proverbs 31:4-5)** Like Satan, alcohol does not show itself as an grotesque looking red monster with horns. That would be very unattractive and appear blatantly deceitful. Rather, it comes as a lovely promise of pleasure and a place of respite from worldly stress. Sensually, it entices with its charm and beauty convincing us that we are deserving, if not entitled, to it's favor. To protect us from Satan's lure, God who always loves us and has only our best interest in mind, warns us to be **"be on the alert"** and to "**be of sober spirit"** so that we will not **"be led astray."**

One of my Stories

It's been my experience, my observation, and my conclusion from studying the literature that alcohol ranks among the top life destroyers. In my personal experience, it degraded my father from an intelligent, athletic, handsome man to a very sad lonely person, finally stealing his life through raising havoc with his body. It told it's lies to my beautiful young son, "be sociable, have a couple beers, you're fine to drive," ending his life way too soon. I swallowed Alcohol's lies, "be normal, have a few drinks, you deserve it," resulting in the lives of my children being turned upside down. As a health care provider, I have sadly listened to multiple renditions of the same song; booze, bar, brawl, jail, and infidelity followed by a chorus of reality and remorse. Though I never drank enough to qualify as even a moderate drinker, I choose to join other healthy and happy people in living a life of sobriety. It gives me the freedom, the physical ability, and the mental clarity to follow the path God has laid out for me with purpose and with joy.

Write Your Story

Standing at another of life's crossroads, you are armed with the truth as presented from multiple perspectives. Will you, with eyes wide open, step up to the high road of sobriety, or will you allow yourself to slide down towards the blinding allure that is the road of alcohol. It is prudent to remain aware that walking the medium between the two roads can prove to be a very slippery slope. If you are skeptical regarding the merits of sobriety, I challenge you to commit yourself to a three month trial in sober living. At the onset and at the three month mark of your venture, evaluate yourself in terms of sleeping, energy level, memory, finances, and any available health metrics such as weight and labs. If you find that you are unable to achieve or to maintain abstinence, know that help is available through Alcoholics Anonymous, Celebrate Recovery, or Substance Abuse Counseling through your physician. During the course of your health venture, you may feel a nudge towards exercising, eating healthier or dropping the nicotine. Feel free to succumb to this nudge as it is an expected positive side effect of sobriety. At the end of your experiment, choose your road, keeping in mind that this is one of those key "the truth will set you free" decisions life presents. Choose wisely my friends.

Epilogue

If after reading these writings it occurs to you that the Bible is demonstrated to be a source of unwavering truth and if you are feeling drawn towards a relationship with the Author, God, consider accepting His open invitation to you. It may be especially compelling to know that He will meet you with open arms right where you are. The following prayer is the Message Bible version of an acceptance of God's invitation, should your heart lead you there. "Dear Lord Jesus, I know that I am a sinner, and I ask for Your forgiveness. I believe You died for my sins and rose from the dead. I turn from my sins and invite You to come into my heart and my life."

REFERENCES

1. Mark Mather Mark, Paola Scommegna , Up to Half of U.S. Premature Deaths are Preventable;Behavioral Key Factors, **National Research Council and Institute of Medicine report**, September 14, 2015
2. W. Mark Mather, Paola Scommegna, Up to Half of U.S. Premature Deaths are Preventable;Behavioral Key Factors, **National Research Council and Institute of Medicine report**, September 14, 2015
3. Corinthians 3:16
4. 1John 1:9
5. Romans 8:28
6. Psalm 46:1
7. Mother Teresa and Mahatma Gandhi
8. Liz Torborg , Getting Enough Vitamin D, Mayo Clinic, March 13, 2018
9. Reinbold Veith, Vitamin Toxicity, Policy and Science, Journal of Bone Mineral Res. 2007
10. Genesis1:3
11. John 8:12
12. Luke 8:16-17
13. Ephesians 4:32
14. Colossians 3:12

15. Genesis 1:29
16. Leviticus 11:46-47
17. Proverbs 25:16
18. Celeste Leigh Pearce, Association Between Life Purpose and Mortality Among U.S. Adults, JAMA Current Open, 5-24-19.
19. Harvard Study, 2017
20. 1Peter 4:10
21. Ephesians 5:15
22. Proverbs 19:21
23. Ephesians 2:10
24. Ercole Vellone et al, Art Improves Stroke Survivors Quality of Life, Health Care in Europe.com, 2-3-2012
25. Genesis 1:31
26. Laurin Eskereis-Winkler, Katherine Milkman et al, A Large Scale Field Experiment Shows Advise Improves Academic Outcomes for the Advisor, Proceedings of the National Academy of Science, 7-8-2019.
27. Steven Post, When Good Things Happen to Bad People, Schocken Books, 1981.
28. Matthew 6:1-4
29. Proverbs 11:25a
30. Benjamin Franklin 1984
31. Matthew 6:1-4
32. Matthew 10:21
33. Psalm 112:5
34. Anne Frank
35. Centers for Disease Control and Prevention, Physical Activity Guidelines for America.
36. Centers for Disease Control and Prevention, Physical Activity Guidelines for America.

37. Proverbs 24:5
38. 2Timothy 4:7
39. 1Corinthians 9:26
40. Kathy Koch PhD, Five to Thrive, Moody, 2-4-2020.
41. Deci and Ryan 2002, Harter 1983
42. Nicole Beurkins, PhD, Holistic Child Psychologist
43. Barry Schlenker, Mike Leary Psychologists
44. Philippians 4:13
45. Ephesians 3:12
46. Philippians 4:13
47. Thomas Edison
48. Genesis. 2:15
49. Psalm 23:2
50. Aristotle
51. Benjamin Franklin
52. Martin Luther King Jr,1957
53. John F. Kennedy, Inaugural Address
54. Sheldon Cohen, Carnegie Mellon University, Psychology in Aging, 6-13-2013
55. Sara Konrath PhD, Andrea Fuhrel-Forbis et al, Volunteering to Help Others Could Lead to Better Health, Journal of Health Psychology, 2012.
56. Acts 20:35
57. Matthew 20:26-28
58. Philippians 2:3-4
59. Ephesians 2:19
60. Mahatma Gandhi
61. Belisa Vranich PhD, Learning the Right Breathing Technique, Learn True Health, 9-25-17.
62. American Lung Association, COPD management tools.
63. Genesis 2:7
64. 2Timothy 3:16-17

65. Nancy Wilson, Bill Bright et al, Use Spiritual Breathing to Surrender Control of Your Life to Christ, Campus Crusade for Christ
66. Luke 23:46
67. Unknown author
68. Margaret Thatcher, former Prime Minister, United Kingdom
69. Theodore Roosevelt
70. Osborne, Moynihan, et al, Married and Co-inhabiting Parents; Relationship Stability, 2007
71. Patrick Moynihan Report
72. Max Lucado, Succeed at Home First, The Teaching Ministry of Max Lucado, 3-2020.
73. Genesis 1:22
74. Ephesians 5:25
75. 1Peter 3:1
76. Ephesians 5:25
77. Proverbs 22:6
78. Matthew 19:19
79. Exodus 20:14
80. 1Timothy 5:8
81. Mark 10:9
82. Mother Teresa
83. Proverbs 17:22
84. Proverbs 15:15
85. Proverbs 25:2
86. Matthew 7:5
87. Stanley Milgram, Seul McCloud et al, the Milgram Shock Experiment, Yale University, 1963
88. Jean Jacque Rousseau
89. John 12:34
90. Ephesians 6:1-3

91. Colossians 3:19
92. Psalm 23:4
93. Luke 11:28
94. Isaiah 41:13
95. World Health Organization
96. Sam Stephens, Washing Hands, Saving Lives: the Surprising Health Benefits of Clean Hands, World Foundation, 10-13-17.
97. Deuteronomy 23:12-14
98. Leviticus 13:47-58
99. Leviticus 13:1
100. Numbers 5:2-4
101. Leviticus 13:45-46
102. Timothy B. Smith, Relationships Improve Your Survival by 50%, Research Finds, Science Daily, Brigham Young, 7-28-10.
103. Dr. Robert Waldinger, Staying Connected, the Secret to Happiness, Harvard Study of Adult Development, 3-28-19.
104. Hebrews 10:24-25
105. Julia Layton, Does Singing Make You Happy?, ISPS, 1998.
106. Ramig, Countryman et al, 1996
107. Ella Fitzgerald
108. Psalm 100:1-2
109. Ephesians 5:19
110. Colossians 3:16
111. Fred Allen
112. Franklin Jones, reporter, humorist
113. Merriam-Webster Dictionary
114. C.S. Lewis
115. Gary Thomas, Sacred Marriage, Zondervan, 2005
116. Deuteronomy 7:7-8

117. 1Corinthians 13:4-5
118. 1John 4:7-8
119. Romans 5:5
120. Proverbs 18:22
121. Ephesians 5:33
122. Water, Essential to your Body, Mayo Clinic, 7-22-20
123. Dr. Stanley Goldfarb, Professor of Medicine, University of Pennsylvania
124. Genesis 1:6-8
125. 1Kings19 4-5
126. Psalm 23:2
127. Matthew 10:42
128. Webster Dictionary
129. Dr. Thomas, Psychologist and Author, Total Life Coaching, WW Norton, 2005.
130. Alcoholics Anonymous, 4th edition Alcoholics Anonymous World Services Inc., 2001
131. Matthew 4:17
132. Matthew 12:34
133. 2Chronicles 7:14
134. Psalm 139:23-24
135. Acts 3:19
136. Nick Foles
137. Winston Churchill
138. 2Timothy 2:5
139. Corinthians 9:25
140. Hebrews 12:1
141. Ken Blanchard, Spencer Johnson, One Minute Manager, William Morrow and Co., 1982
142. Carol Dweck PhD, Encouragement Breaks Down Barriers, Sanford University, 11-2007.
143. Proverbs 18:21

144. Luke 6:38
145. Unknown six year old student
146. Stephen King
147. Health Benefits of Vacations, Framingham Study, 2014.
148. University of Vienna Study, Pub Med, 4-2000.
149. Changes in well-being with time away from work, Project Time Off.
150. Sixty minute nap is good for the memory, Adult Health Napping do's and don'ts, Mayo Clinic.
151. Alexandro Leeras, why you need to Stop Thinking You are too busy to Take Breaks, University of Illinois, 9-2-2014.
152. Exodus 20:8-19
153. Matthew 11:28-30
154. Psalm 23:1-5
155. Alcoholics Anonymous, 4th edition Alcoholics Anonymous World Services Inc., 2001
156. Alcoholics Anonymous, 4th edition Alcoholics Anonymous World Services Inc., 2001
157. Matthew 18:21-22
158. Matthew 6:12
159. Philippians
160. Albert Einstein
161. McGill University, Neuro Chemistry Music Study
162. Ephesians 5:19
163. Warren Buffett
164. Danielle Kassow, Thrive by Five, C.J. Dunst, 2008.
165. Melissa Koenig, Paul Harris, Trust in Testimony, Pub Med Research, 10-01-2004.
166. Russell Barkley, Child Psychologist, Life Stages of Trust, 9-1-2008.

167. 7 Ways to Build Trust in a Relationship, Psychology Today, 12-12-2018.
168. Ernest Hemmingway
169. Jerry Bridges, Trusting God, Nav Press, 2008
170. Isaiah 55:8-9
171. Romans 8:28
172. Proverbs 3:5-8
173. Herbert Benson M.D., Mind/Body Institute, Enhancing Health Through Body/Mind Healing, Harvard Medical School, 9-10-12.
174. Galileo
175. Joshua 1:8
176. Philippians 4:7
177. Philippians 4:13
178. Carl Jung
179. Adult Health Denial: When it Helps; When it Hurts, Mayo Clinic
180. Alcoholics Anonymous, 4th edition Alcoholics Anonymous World Services Inc., 2001
181. Amy Morin, Psychotherapist, Healthy Coping Skills for Uncomfortable Emotions, 4-3-20.
182. C.S. Lewis
183. Psalm 46:10
184. Matthew 22:36-40
185. Galatians 3:28
186. Romans 2:11
187. Revelation 7:9-10
188. Psalm 139:23
189. Dog Ownership After a Major Cardiovascular Event, Swedish Study, 10-08-2019.
190. Owning a Dog Linked to Healthier Heart and Longer Life, Meta Analysis 70 years, 2019.

191. Pet Therapy: Animals as Healers, Mayo Clinic Staff, Mayo Clinic
192. Genesis 2:18-19
193. Genesis 1:28
194. Exodus 20:9-11
195. Exodus 23:12
196. Robert Feldman, The Liar in Your Life, 8-4-2009.
197. Abraham Lincoln
198. Proverbs 12:22
199. Psalm 85:12
200. Mischel, Chae Mamayek et al, Self Control as Self Regulation: A Return to Control Theory, Journal of Deviant Behavior 2014, Vol 38, 2017.
201. Alder, Disadvantage, Self Control, and Health, National Academy of Sciences of USA, 2015.
202. Seligman, It's Time: A Meta-Analysis on the Self-Control Deviance Link, Journal of Criminal Justice, 2-20-2017.
203. Miller et al, Motivating the Unmotivated: How Health Behavior Can be Changed in Those Unwilling to Change, Frontiers in Psychology, 6-16-2015.
204. Galatians 5:22-23
205. 2Timothy 1:7
206. 1Corinthians 10:13
207. Cambridge Dictionary
208. Cambridge Dictionary
209. The Denial of Reality, Psychology Today, 12-08-2015.
210. Wayne Riggs, Open Mindedness, Metaphilosophy, 1-11-2020.
211. Aristotle
212. John 8:32

213. Proverbs 18:2
214. Webster's Dictionary
215. Romans 1:18-19
216. C.S. Lewis
217. Stewart Wolpert, Putting Feelings into Words Produces Therapeutic Effects in the Brain, UCLA newsroom, 6-21-2007.
218. Can Helping Your Todo's Help You Doze?, Baylor University Sleep Neuroscience and Cognition Lab, 1-11-2018.
219. Christina Karns, Inspire Altruism Through an Attitude of Gratitude, University of Oregon Research, 12-14-2017.
220. Terry Goodrich, Baylor University Sleep Neuroscience and Cognition Lab
221. James Pennebaker, Psychologist and Researcher,University of Texas @ Austin
222. Anne Frank
223. Jeremiah 30:2
224. Psalm 119:15
225. William Wordsworth
226. Proverbs 3:5-6
227. Psalm 18:2
228. Matthew 11:28-29
229. Psalm 127:2
230. Calvin Coolidge
231. Albert Einstein
232. Martin Luther King Jr.
233. Jean Weichai, M.D., The Neuroscience of Perseverance, Psychology Today, 12-26-2011.
234. Romans 5:3-5
235. Philippians 3:14

236. Ronald Riggio PhD, There is Magic in Your Smile; How Smiling Affects Your Brain, Psychology Today, 6-25-2012.
237. Thich Nhat Hanh, Zen Master.
238. Matthew 11:19
239. Proverbs 17:22
240. Proverbs 31:25
241. Jill Shalvis, quote, author of Simply Irresistible.
242. Webster's Dictionary
243. Charles Snyder et al, Psychologists, The Hope Theory, 1991.
244. Jerry Groopman, Anatomy of Hope, Random House, 01-11-2005.
245. Pastor Rick Warren, Why Hope Isn't the Same as Optimism, Daily Hope, 5-2-17.
246. Romans 15:13
247. Matthew 6:32-33
248. Chinese Proverb
249. Webster's Dictionary
250. Webster's Dictionary
251. Jim Stone, Understanding Impatience, Psychology Today, 11-4-2014.
252. Schnitker and Emmons, An Examination of Patience and Well-Being, Research Gate, 2007.
253. Jim Stone PhD, Take a Deep Breath, Psychology Today, 7-29-16.
254. Galatians 5:22
255. Timothy 4:2
256. Pastor Charles Stanley, Developing Patience, In Touch Crosswalk.com, 4-27-2012.
257. 2Timothy 2:24
258. Ecclesiastes 7:9
259. Socrates

260. Erik Erikson, Theory of Psychosocial Development, Humble ISD.net.
261. Althea Young PhD
262. Genesis 1:27
263. Carolyn Gregoire, Why Finding Time Each Day for Creativity Makes You Happier, the New Zealand Study, Huffpost.com, 12-2-2016.
264. Heather Stuckney, The Connection Between Art, Healing, and Public Health, American Journal of Public Health, 9-20-2011.
265. How Does Art Affect the Brain, Harvard Medical School, 11-20-2017.
266. Genesis 1:1.
267. Genesis 1:27
268. 1Timothy 4:14-15
269. Colossians 3:23
270. Ursula Leguin, The Creative Adult is the Child Who Survived, Create Space, 8-18-18.
271. Richard Wagner, composer, quote.
272. Merriam-Webster Dictionary
273. J.D. Salinger, author, quote.
274. Ken Kers, PhD, 7 Qualities of a Joyful PersonUnited Kingdom Study, UK Study, 2019.
275. 1Peter 4:10
276. 1John 1-4
277. Rick Warren, The Purpose Driven Life, Zondervan, 2002.
278. Psalm 40:4
279. Alcoholics Anonymous, 4th edition Alcoholics Anonymous World Services Inc., 2001
280. Mark Twain
281. Willie Nelson

282. Summer Allen PhD, The Science of Gratitude, Greater Good Science Center at the U.S. Berkley, May 2018.
283. Philippians 4:6-7
284. 1Thessalonians 5:16-18
285. Michael Kraft M.D., psychologist at Grace Counseling in Denver, Mistress of the Universe: Learning to Let Go of Control, Focus on the Family, 1-1-2003.
286. Alcoholics Anonymous, 4th edition Alcoholics Anonymous World Services Inc., 2001
287. Alcoholics Anonymous, 4th edition Alcoholics Anonymous World Services Inc., 2001
288. Seymour, Tice et al, Article in Psychology of Religion and Spirituality, Psychology Today, 5-20-12.
289. If Our Surrender is to God, it Tends to Be Associated with Lower Reported Stress. Mayo Clinic.
290. Ann Landers
291. 1Peter 5:7
292. Psalm 34:17
293. Matthew 27:50
294. Matthew 6:9-13
295. Alcoholics Anonymous, 4th edition Alcoholics Anonymous World Services Inc., 2001
296. Eckhardt Toile
297. Robert Wood Johnson Foundation Publication, March 2013
298. Mental Health Effects of Long Hours, Night and Week-end Work, and Short Rest Periods, Social Sciences and Medicine, Feb. 2020.

299. E.B. Faragher, M. Cass et al, A large scale meta analysis of almost 500 studies, Strong Relationshio Between Job Satisfaction and Mental Health.
300. Genesis 1:28
301. 2Thessalonians 3:10
302. Colossians 3:23
303. James 1:5
304. Leviticus 19:34
305. Hebrews 13:2
306. Alfred Tennyson, quote.
307. C.S. Lewis
308. Merriam-Webster
309. Rick Pitino, quote.
310. Matthew 20:28
311. James 4:6
312. Philippians 2:3-5
313. Matthew 5:8
314. Proverbs 25:14
315. Confucius
316. Tim Tebow
317. Aristotle
318. Mark 1:35
319. Exodus 20:8-11
320. Daniel 6:10
321. Proverbs 21:5
322. Psalm 24:1-2
323. Buddha
324. Jacqueline Carter, Rasmus, et al, How Mindful Are You, Harvard Business Review, 3-29-17.
325. Pastor Rick Warren, Don't Be Afraid, Daily Hope, 4-28-16.
326. Matthew 6:34

327. 1John 1:98
328. Hebrews 8:12
329. Mark Twain
330. Dietary Guidelines for Americans, Center for Disease Control, American Dietary Association, American Dietary Association, 2015-2020.
331. Proverbs 20:1
332. 1Peter5:8-9
333. Romans 13:13
334. Ephesians 5:18
335. Proverbs 31:4-5

Endorsements

After reading just a couple of Path to Health chapters, (Where Science Meets Scripture), I thought.... hmmmm..she may be onto something. Can it really be that simple. As a matter of fact ...yes it can. Water, smiling, sunshine, all such simple everyday concepts but as it turns out they were all part of the plan. The Bible, as Susan realized, suggested all of these as ways to a healthier life. Now, medicine is coming around to the same conclusions. Instead of taking pills , making some adjustments to our daily lives can make a world of difference. Susan has made some legitimate points. I can not possibly apply them all at once, but I have certainly been motivated to take some "baby steps" toward better spiritual and physical health.

Patricia White, Retired RDH

After reading Susan's chapter on "Singing", it affirmed what I thought I knew. I knew singing made me feel better, made me feel lighter, made me less anxious and depressed but reading the correlation between singing and brain function reinforced it all. Then to think of singing as a means of prayer made the picture complete! When I sing in the grocery store or car, I feel lit up inside; when I sing in church, I feel lifted up in prayer. No matter the circumstances, prayerful singing is a joyous sound! Singing psalms and the unleashing of all of the happy chemicals in my brain helps to make me healthy in body and soul!

Anna Audioun, Retired Victims Advocate

What I enjoyed about this book that Susan has written is the alignment she has created. She has aligned medical science, God's Word the Bible, her own experiences and how you can, step by step, accomplish the development of these habits for your own physical, emotional, and spiritual health. Do you want to think better, feel better and know that this is the kind of life that the creator of our human bodies and minds had intended for us all along?? Every time I read Susan's weekly offering, by the end of it, I would always think "everyone needs to read this", "I wish everyone could read this", "wouldn't it be nice if every person who graduated from high school read this or every new bride and groom needs to read this!!!" I was always blown away! This book helps you build wisdom for the way you are supposed to live, the habits you would want to form, so the choices you make are for good physical, emotional and spiritual health which will lead to a happier, healthier life. Louise Desare

It is without reservation that I recommend Susan Goe's "Path to Health (Where Science Meets Scripture) !" In the spirit of full disclosure, she is my big sister. That doesn't mean her book isn't brilliant. The structure is particularly valuable. She starts with "What Science Says" then moves to "What God Says" (amazingly consistent!). The next section is one of her stories and she finally suggests the reader write their own story. My favorite chapter may be the one on "Open Minded." The whole idea that we children of God are free to think about anything and everything is liberating. She manages to mention me and Aristotle in the same essay. That's talent. In this chapter she describes a hypothetical conversation with a child who may be making a sketchy decision. After saying a quick prayer she says to "listen, listen, listen" and then converse. Although she doesn't use the term, that's the Socratic method in spades. Science, the Greek philosophers, and God all wrapped up in one brief dissertation. That's what I call "inspired."

Join my sister on her adventure. John White, Registered Respiratory Therapist

About the Author

Susan Goe is the author of one other book, *Shining My Light*, written under a pseudonym, "Gee". *Shining My Light* was written as her testimony to her family so that they might benefit from lessons learned from her life journey. Shortly after the publication of *Shining My Light*, she was strongly inspired to address a wider audience, those seeking genuine health. After fifty years as a health care provider, she became disillusioned with the medical model to provide true health. She was beginning to realize that, if there were a better system, it would need to consider the whole person; their physical, their emotional and their spiritual selves. It was after years of studying scripture, while simultaneously practicing medicine, that a connection was made and the light went on. Science, at that time, had advanced to the point where it's gold standards for health were synchronizing with those recorded in the bible for over two thousand years. Her writings suggest pragmatic life strategies towards true health that is supported by both science and scripture. Her hearts desire is for her readers to not only achieve health and happiness but to be drawn towards a relationship with God.

CPSIA information can be obtained
at www.ICGtesting.com
Printed in the USA
LVHW072038261020
669863LV00008B/113